The Caregiver's Guide to
Memory Care and Dementia Communities

A JOHNS HOPKINS PRESS HEALTH BOOK

THE *Caregiver's Guide* TO

Memory Care and Dementia Communities

Rachael Wonderlin

Foreword by Michelle Tristani

Johns Hopkins University Press | *Baltimore*

© 2022 Johns Hopkins University Press
All rights reserved. Published 2022
Printed in the United States of America on acid-free paper
2 4 6 8 9 7 5 3

Johns Hopkins University Press
2715 North Charles Street
Baltimore, Maryland 21218-4363
www.press.jhu.edu

Library of Congress Cataloging-in-Publication Data

Names: Wonderlin, Rachael, 1989– author.
Title: The caregiver's guide to memory care and dementia communities / Rachael Wonderlin ; foreword by Michelle Tristani.
Description: Baltimore : Johns Hopkins University Press, 2022. | Series: A Johns Hopkins Press health book | Includes index.
Identifiers: LCCN 2021053773 | ISBN 9781421444321 (paperback) | ISBN 9781421444338 (ebook)
Subjects: LCSH: Dementia—Handbooks, manuals, etc. | Dementia—Patients—Care—Handbooks, manuals, etc. | Caregivers—Handbooks, manuals, etc. | Long-term care facilities.
Classification: LCC RC521 .W626 2022 | DDC 616.8/3—dc23/eng/20211124 ;
LC record available at https://lccn.loc.gov/2021053773

A catalog record for this book is available from the British Library.

Special discounts are available for bulk purchases of this book. For more information, please contact Special Sales at specialsales@jh.edu.

For everyone who has been reading my blog posts, books, listening to my podcast, watching my videos, and engaging with me for years.

For everyone who ever felt like they were shouldering this burden alone.

I'm glad you're here. It is the gift of a lifetime to be able to provide you with some support and, hopefully, some comfort. Thank you.

Contents

Foreword, by Michelle Tristani   ix

PART I Defining and Understanding Dementia   1

1. Why This Book Is Worth Reading   3
2. What Is Dementia?   6
3. Causes of Dementia   13

4. Stages of Dementia   20
5. Medications   26

PART II Communicating with People Living with Dementia   33

6. Embracing Someone's Reality   35
7. Why Logic, Quizzing, and Reorientation Don't Work   41
8. Yes, and … : Improvisation and Dementia   47
9. Communicating with Someone Experiencing Hallucinations and Delusions   52

10. Helping with Timeline Confusion   58
11. Personal Preferences   63
12. Becoming a Dementia Detective   69
13. Aphasia   78

PART III Caregiver Stress and Choosing a Care Community   85

14. Caregiving Stress   87
15. Guilt and Taking Things Away   94
16. How to Handle Family Dynamics When Choosing a Care Community   101
17. Myths about Care Communities   107

18. At-Home Safety   112
19. When Is It Time to Move Your Loved One?   117
20. What Types of Communities Exist?   124
21. Cost of Care   132

PART IV Caregiving in a Care Community   139

22. What to Expect at a Dementia
Care Community   141

23. Move-In Day   148

24. Remember That Caregiving
Is an Imperfect Science   154

25. Visiting and Saying Goodbye   160

26. Day Trips and Outings   166

27. Activities   171

28. Building a Dementia-Friendly
Environment   179

PART V Changes in Care   185

29. When Technology Works and
When It Doesn't   187

30. When It's Time for a Dietary
Change   192

31. Friendships and Disagreements
among Residents   199

32. Sex and Sexual Orientation   205

33. When It's Time for Hospice   214

34. When There's a Hospital Trip   220

35. Final Thoughts and Notes   225

Appendix. Clinical Dementia Rating Scale   231
Index   237

Foreword

Michelle Tristani

Rachael Wonderlin's approach to training and coaching in the memory care arena is entirely refreshing, exceptionally fun, and extremely practical. She provides "dementia training with an attitude." Her new book is a comprehensive collection of positive insights and interventions for everyone who supports individuals living with dementia.

The approach described in this book reflects a significant paradigm shift in dementia care, changing the perspective from negative to positive, from disability to ability. Memory care is not what you think it is; it is what you think it is not. Memory care is not only about cognitive testing or brain imaging. It does not have to be about losing oneself or giving up or feeling alone. It is not about being cared *for* but being cared *about*; it is not about "what is the matter with us" but "what matters to us." It is all about connecting to what is most important at each stage of dementia. It is about capturing and developing preserved abilities, about setting up the environment for success, and about focusing on the possibilities.

If you are confused about persons that are confused, you are not alone. With so many varied causes of dementia, abundant new research, and the substantial impact of COVID-19 on the progression of all neurodegenerative diagnoses, it is understandable to be overwhelmed.

This book begins by outlining commonly used terms and answers frequently asked questions. In this way, we are positioned to dive into more complex topics with a consistent foundation.

Rachael hints at ways in which we must counter ageism as she outlines the negative connotation via the use of the label "senility" and other ageist terms. Throughout the book, dementia case studies offer an empathetic perspective and are written from the point of view of the person living with dementia. The connections these case studies provide are among the most valuable insights in Rachael's book.

Step by step, we are guided through the process of Embracing Their Reality. This is truly a lesson in mindfulness and centering ourselves first as we work to differentially diagnose our reality versus the reality of the person with dementia. Once we determine where the person is in their reality and timeline, we then can make a true and strong connection. This connection leads to building trust within the relationship. It is trust that diffuses anxiety, frustration, fear, and feelings of loss of control within the person living with dementia.

The use of the term *frontline* has become commonplace since the start of the COVID-19 pandemic. All chapters focus on the skill of frontline community care partners. At the close of each chapter, "Putting It into Practice" sections assist us in applying the tools, individualized skills, and plans in the course of daily caregiving. Rachael keeps it real with typical life situations that maximize our ability to immediately put new skills into practice. Each chapter builds upon the next for a cumulative increase in our confidence and skill readiness.

I am a believer of approaching challenges without regrets. Dementia is a challenge to say the least. As we read and review the guidance and reassurance Rachael provides, our confidence increases. Making meaningful connections throughout each day profoundly affects our lives, the lives of persons living with dementia, and the lives of all those watching us turn dementia care communication around.

Michelle Tristani, MS/CCC-SLP, is a cognitive disorders and dementia specialist as well as a national leader, coach, and trainer in dementia care.

PART I

Defining and Understanding Dementia

I begin this book with necessary information about what dementia is and why an accurate diagnosis is so important. I also introduce some key terms used throughout the book. Information about the medications for treating dementia can be found in chapter 5. Although I am not a physician, I do provide an overview of certain medications and how they are used so that you can discuss the options with your loved one's doctor and health care team. It is important to discuss diagnosis, prognosis, staging, treatment, and other relevant issues with a medical professional who is knowledgeable about dementia.

CHAPTER 1

Why This Book Is Worth Reading

I love working in the field of dementia care. My goal, through my blog, podcast, books, and live workshops, is to provide caregivers with useful skills. By this I mean actions you can take today, immediately, based on your needs in caring for someone living with dementia. I truly believe that's the whole point of learning—to gain skills and education that you can put into practice.

Most chapters in this book conclude with a Putting It into Practice section.

Some of these sections contain a set of questions for you to answer. Others are assignments to complete, thoughts to consider, or tips for honing a new skill. These aren't mandatory (of course), but I hope that you will think of them as a way to expand the discussion we are having throughout this book. I have also included resources at the end of each chapter, such as websites, books, and products for purchase that I have utilized with success.

Definitions

I have written this book for caregivers. Who is a caregiver? If you are reading this, the answer is you! *Anyone who cares for someone living with dementia, in any capacity, paid or unpaid, can be called a caregiver or care partner.* Caregivers are often related to the person living with dementia, and those caregivers are rarely paid for this work. It is truly a labor of love. Note that being a care partner does not necessarily mean you need to be with the person living with dementia twenty-four hours a day, seven days a week.

What is long-term care? *Long-term care includes services and communities that cater to aging adults.* The many types of long-term care include in-home care, assisted living, personal care, skilled nursing, long-term nursing care, respite care, adult day care, continuing care retirement communities (CCRCs), dementia care communities, and memory care communities.

We will discuss the various communities in chapter 20. For the moment, it is important to understand that long-term care is not just one type of care. Many caregivers feel like their choices for care for a loved one are limited to in-home care or a nursing home. Fortunately, though, there are many options. I have also found that many families are unclear what a nursing home really is, and that many people refer to assisted living communities as "nursing homes."

What is dementia? *Dementia is an umbrella term for a group of diseases that are characterized by the loss of cognitive function over time.* Alzheimer disease is the most common form of dementia. Many people think that the only form of dementia is Alzheimer disease. But let's compare it to another well-known set of diseases. If you find out that a person you know has cancer, you'll probably ask, "What type of cancer?" because there are many different types of cancer. Similarly, dementia can result from various diseases. Dementia is not a part of normal aging. Many people know older adults who are "sharp as a tack." There are more than a hundred different causes of dementia, all of which exhibit different symptoms and affect the brain in different ways.

You just read that dementia diseases cause cognitive decline. But what is cognitive decline? *Cognitive decline is the reduction in function over time of memory, speech, movement, thinking, and reasoning.* Symptoms of cognitive decline can include:

- difficulty making decisions
- forgetting important dates
- slowed reaction time when driving
- slowed movement
- delayed speech
- poor judgment in social situations
- trouble remembering names

and much more.

People with dementia may have difficulty with the activities of daily living (ADLs), such as bathing, dressing, grooming, toileting, eating, and walking. They may have trouble with more challenging tasks, such as sending an e-mail, writing a check, doing laundry, or cooking. These complex tasks are usually referred to as *instrumental activities of daily living,* or IADLs. Sometimes a person with dementia will experience personality changes, sudden mood swings, and hallucinations. The types of cognitive decline that people living with dementia encounter are wide and varied.

I regularly use the term *dementia care community.* What is a dementia care community (DCC)? *DCCs are places that host adults living with dementia.* A DCC could be several wings or a unit within a larger community, or it could be a stand-alone community. A DCC could even be an adult day care center that caters to people living with dementia. Oftentimes, dementia care communities are known as memory care communities. DCCs differ from other types of communities in a few key ways. Unlike other long-term care communities, dementia-care-specific communities cater to those living with dementia. Residents of assisted living facilities (ALFs) do not necessarily have dementia—although they can—and are typically more physically and cognitively able than adults in skilled nursing facilities (SNFs) or dementia care communities. Residents in nursing homes are usually there either for short-term rehabilitation or are almost entirely physically dependent on others for care. Sometimes, in the last stages of dementia, as they become more physically dependent, residents will move from dementia care to a long-term-care nursing home. More often, however, they will live in the dementia care community until death. Before choosing a dementia care community, ask the community's administrator what happens as a resident's dementia progresses.

Are hospice and palliative care programs available to assist in resident care? Do most residents pass away at the community? These important questions will help you learn more about a dementia care community's policies, procedures, and assistance as a loved one is dying. We will dive deeper into this subject in later chapters. In chapter 2, we review what dementia is and how one would go about getting a diagnosis.

Putting It into Practice

In this first activity, let's ask some "big" questions. My hope is that we will have thoroughly answered all these questions, and more, by the last page of this book.

1. What is my first question about dementia?

_____

2. What is the difference between dementia and Alzheimer disease?

_____

3. What is my biggest concern about my loved one living with dementia?

_____

4. What is my goal in reading this book? What do I hope to learn?

_____

RESOURCES

Alzheimer's Association. 2021. Understanding Alzheimer's Disease and Dementia. https://www.alz.org/alzheimer_s_dementia.

Mace, N. L., and P. V. Rabins. 2021. *The 36-Hour Day: A Family Guide to Caring for People Who* *Have Alzheimer Disease and Other Dementias*, 7th ed. Baltimore: Johns Hopkins University Press.

National Institutes of Aging. 2021. Alzheimer's Disease and Related Dementias. https://www.nia.nih.gov/health/alzheimers.

CHAPTER 2

What Is Dementia?

Avoiding confusion about dementia, Alzheimer disease, and related conditions

When people hear "dementia," they think of two things: memory loss and Alzheimer disease. I am regularly asked, "What is the difference between dementia and Alzheimer disease?" In this chapter, we dive into the myths and misunderstandings that surround dementia. This is important, because for us to provide the best possible care for someone living with dementia, we first need to understand what it is.

As noted in chapter 1, dementia is not one disease; it is a group of symptoms caused by more than a hundred different diseases. Alzheimer disease is one among those hundred or so diseases. The difference between dementia and Alzheimer disease is like the difference between cancer and skin cancer: one is the umbrella term, and the other is an actual disease. This is why, for most of this book, I write "dementia" instead of "Alzheimer disease" or any other form of cognitive loss. Dr. Peter V. Rabins in his book *Is It Alzheimer's?* defines what dementia is.

Dementia is any disease that has these four characteristics.

1. Onset begins in adulthood
2. There is a decline in two or more aspects of thinking

3. There is a decline in daily function due to these thinking impairments
4. A person still has normal levels of alertness and concentration

What defines a "decline in thinking"? A decline in thinking can include difficulty with memory, language, perception, judgment, and organization of information (Rabins, p. 4)

The latest edition of the *Diagnostic and Statistical Manual of Mental Disorders (DSM)* effectively changes the word *dementia* to *neurocognitive disorder*, or NCD. The *DSM* divides NCDs into mild and major neurocognitive disorders. Alzheimer disease can be categorized as both mild NCD (early stages of Alzheimer disease) and major NCD (later stages of Alzheimer disease). According to the website Psychiatry Online, "Although cognitive deficits are present in many if not all mental disorders (e.g., schizophrenia, bipolar disorders), only disorders whose core features are cognitive are included in the NCD category. The NCDs are those in which impaired cognition has not been present since birth or very early life, and thus represents a decline from a previously attained level of functioning." Because the term is relatively new, neurocognitive disorder has not yet made its way into common usage.

Symptoms of Dementia

In chapter 1, I defined *cognitive decline* as the reduction in function over time of memory, speech, movement, thinking, and reasoning. Among the symptoms of cognitive decline is short-term memory impairment. People living with dementia also develop difficulty with their *activities of daily living* (ADLs), such as bathing, dressing, grooming, toileting, eating, and walking. They will eventually have trouble with more challenging tasks, such as sending an email, writing a check, cooking, cleaning, and doing laundry. These complex tasks are usually referred to as *instrumental activities of daily living*, or IADLs. Sometimes a person with dementia will experience personality changes, sudden mood swings, or visual or auditory hallucinations. The types of cognitive decline that people with dementia encounter are wide and varied.

Dementia almost always worsens and eventually leads to death. Only about 1% of dementias are reversible. An example of a reversible dementia is one caused by a vitamin deficiency. Although different dementias affect the brain in physiologically different ways, all dementias repeatedly damage the brain until it stops working, and the body shuts down. You might have heard of a person with dementia who died in a choking incident or a fall. In truth, their dementia likely caused them to choke or fall. If the person had not been impaired by dementia, they likely would have known what to do if they were choking or might have avoided falling.

Myths about Dementia

Historically, the words "senile" and "senility" were used to refer to dementia, when someone didn't know what the actual problem was. When I hear someone use these words to describe someone with dementia, I let them know that these are "bad words" in my field, because they have a negative and pejorative connotation. You may have also heard a phrase like "hardening of the arteries" when someone was talking about a loved one's dementia diagnosis. A friend may have described another individual as "just getting old" or "elderly" when describing their memory impairment. We prefer not to use these words or phrases any longer in the field of geriatrics. Instead we use "dementia" and "aging."

Dementia is not a part of normal aging, although the chance of getting dementia increases as you age. Many people encounter some natural age-related changes in cognition, such as the ability to recall names with ease. Most experts agree that if you are concerned about your cognition or the cognition of a loved one, it is best to have a medical workup that attempts to find the cause.

Sometimes families fear that because a relative has dementia the rest of the family is also at risk for developing the disease. "If a parent or sibling has clinically diagnosed Alzheimer disease, then your risk of developing Alzheimer disease is two and a half to three times more likely than someone whose parents and siblings did not develop Alzheimer disease," writes Dr. Peter Rabins (p. 67). Another cause of dementia is environmental. We know that one gene associated with Alzheimer disease is called the apolipoprotein E gene, or APOE gene (Mayo Clinic website). Genes come in different "flavors" that we call alleles. Every person has two copies of a gene. So, you can have two of the same allele or two different alleles of a gene. It depends on what your parents have and what they passed on to you. The APOE gene has three common forms. If a person has one copy of the APOE e4 allele, then their risk of developing Alzheimer disease rises to 35%. Looking at the entire population, the overall risk for developing dementia by age 80 is between 15% and 35% (Rabins, p. 66).

Early-onset or younger-onset dementia is dementia that starts before the age of 65, sometimes as early as in a person's thirties. So far, researchers have identified three genes that when mutated cause younger-onset Alzheimer disease. Fortunately, younger-onset Alzheimer disease is rare (Rabins, p. 66).

Dementia is much more than just a memory problem. Although many dementia care communities are called memory care units, it's quite possible that a number of the individuals living there do not have significant memory problems. Residents that I have worked with in dementia care communities have mental and physical symptoms, such as loss of reasoning, inability to make safe decisions, trouble walking, difficulty speaking, inability to bathe independently, and many more.

Since dementia is not just one disease, it is useful to determine the cause of someone's dementia. Often, a person will say, "My mom has dementia" and leave it at that, because they do not realize there is a lot more information they could gather about their mother's disease. They might be saying that mom has dementia because they have noticed that she has some memory loss or other types of cognitive decline. But some causes of cognitive impairments are reversible (for example, operable brain tumors), so it is imperative that your family member or friend receives a full medical workup. True forms of dementia affect a person's ability to function both physically and mentally over time. A person can have more than one form of dementia at the same time.

Let's turn back to our opening question: "What is the difference between Alzheimer disease and dementia?" To be clear, Alzheimer disease *is* dementia. Alzheimer disease is the most common form of cognitive decline in older adults, so it gets more attention than other dementias.

Currently, there aren't any medications that stop or prevent dementia. But there are medications that can help alleviate symptoms of dementia and in some cases even slow the progression of cognitive decline. We will look at this in a lot more detail in chapter 5.

What Isn't Dementia?

There are numerous conditions that share some symptoms with dementia but are not dementia. How do we tell them apart? For one, dementia and delirium are not the same thing. *Delirium* is a sudden onset of confusion, and it is often reversible. Delirium can be caused by many different medical issues, such as an adverse medication interaction, fall, stroke, or urinary tract infection. I often tell families of people living with dementia that dementia does not get dramatically worse overnight. This means that if you are visiting someone who is significantly more confused and agitated than they were the day before, it is advisable that they undergo a medical evaluation. Delirium caused by a urinary tract infection, stroke, medication interaction, or fall can temporarily exacerbate someone's dementia.

A condition often referred to as *sundowning* is also not a form of dementia, although it can be a symptom of dementia. In a way, every one of us "sundowns," that is, as the day wears on, we sometimes grow tired and become more agitated or irritable. This does not happen to everyone with dementia, and it does not happen every day. In fact, it does not have to be correlated with the sun, although it often is.

Mild cognitive impairment is also not dementia, nor is it considered normal age-related cognitive decline. Mild cognitive impairment (MCI) is cognitive function that is below the mean for that individual's age, such as a decline between 30% and 45% in memory or another cognitive function. People living with MCI will often progress to a form of dementia. Some people, however, stay the same or improve, returning to a normal level of cognition. People living with MCI can usually live independently and manage their daily tasks, but they may have difficulty remembering appointments or names (Rabins, p. 8).

How Do You Get Tested for Dementia?

Most experts agree that it's important to determine whether someone has dementia early on in the disease process. If you are thinking, "If there's no cure, what's the point?" you aren't alone; many people feel the same way. My response is, getting an early diagnosis helps you to plan accordingly. Planning for your family may mean drawing up a will or starting discussions about plans for future home care or move to a dementia care community. An early diagnosis also gives you more information about what the cause of your friend's dementia may be. Since there are many different causes of dementia, there is a good deal of variability in the symptoms you may see. It helps to know what symptoms to expect in that person's disease progression.

How do you or a loved one get tested for dementia? A lot of people opt solely for a visit to their family physician, but if possible, it is best to see a team of professionals that specializes in dementia, or a neurologist or geriatrician with advanced knowledge about cognitive impairments. Some hospitals, such as the Penn Memory Center, part of the University of Pennsylvania Health System in Philadelphia, offer programs that provide families with full medical and neuropsychological workups. Here is a breakdown of the type of testing that occurs at a hospital like the Penn Memory Center.

If you are the person being tested for dementia:

- You may be required to make two visits to the testing site. At Penn Memory Center, the new-patient experience consists of two appointments: one that is an initial comprehensive evaluation totaling ninety minutes, and another four to six weeks later totaling sixty minutes.

- You'll be asked to bring a family member or friend with you to the testing site.
- During the first visit, a social worker will do an intake interview, including asking a few questions about your current health and well-being.
- You will be seen by a psychometric tester, who will thoroughly test your memory and cognitive functions with written, drawn, and spoken exams.
- You, your physician, and friend or family member will meet to go over the preliminary findings of the visit. The doctors might order brain imaging before the next visit.
- Between the first and second visit, the center receives your brain imaging results and looks over the results of the cognitive testing.
- During the second visit, the physician and a social worker review the results of all the testing and explain the diagnosis and how it was reached. They might outline a health care plan or a plan for future visits (Penn Memory Center).

If you are the family member or care partner:

- A social worker will ask in-depth questions about you and the person living with dementia. They will ask about your relationship, your family history, their family history, and age or date of potential dementia onset. Be prepared that some of these questions could be stressful, depending on your relationship with the person who has dementia.
- You will also see the psychiatrist. They will ask about the person's change in condition, their back-

ground, their mood, and their level of insight into their own condition.

- The nurse practitioner or physician assistant will sort through their medications, so make sure you bring an updated list of all their medications. They will probably ask you a few questions, as well.
- You may meet with another team member who will talk to you about resources and support groups in the area.

This team-based approach to diagnosis is comprehensive and the best you could ask for when it comes to getting an accurate diagnosis. You might not have a program like this in your area, or perhaps the waitlist for the program is far too long. The next best approach is to find a geriatrician or neurologist who specializes in aging. They will know what types of tests to do and what to look for. This seems obvious, but it's important. I have had care partners tell me that their regular doctors "missed" a loved one's dementia diagnosis because they "weren't looking for it." Think of it this way: if you are a cardiologist, are you necessarily looking at a patient's cognitive status as well as their cardiovascular issue? Consider, too, that physicians may miss a patient's dementia when the patient can still speak fluently about their physical health, the weather, and basic topics that come up during the exam.

In chapter 3, we review what some of the main causes of cognitive decline actually are and how to distinguish among them. Even though the material and concepts are challenging, it's helpful to understand that there are many causes of dementia and that a person can have a multitude of symptoms.

Putting It into Practice

One great recommendation for anyone considering having their loved one tested for dementia (and for people in general) is to document their medical history in a list that you can share with the doctor. Preparing this list in advance can save you time and make the visit less stressful.

The list can include the following:

Medical history
Have they been diagnosed with any conditions? List them.

_____

Have they been hospitalized? If so, what for and on what date(s)?

_____

Have they ever been diagnosed with COVID-19?

_____

Have they been vaccinated for COVID-19? Include the date(s) of vaccination, along with which vaccine they received.

_____

Family history
Do their immediate family members have any health conditions we should know about?

_____

Medications
What medications are they taking? Please be specific and include the dose and how often they take the specific drug.

_____

Supplements
List any supplements they may take, such as teas, herbs, vitamins, and so forth. Supplements sometimes interact with other medications.

_____

What brings them to the doctor?

_____

Any other concerns you or your loved one want to mention?

_____

RESOURCES

DSM Library at Psychiatry Online. 2021. Neurocognitive Disorders. https://dsm .psychiatryonline.org/doi/abs/10.1176/appi .books.9780890425596.dsm17.

Mayo Clinic. 2021. Alzheimer's Genes: Are You at Risk? https://www.mayoclinic .org/diseases-conditions/alzheimers -disease/in-depth/alzheimers-genes/art -20046552.

Penn Memory Center. 2019. Patient Care. https:// pennmemorycenter.org/patient-care.

Rabins, P. V. 2020. _Is It Alzheimer's? 101 Answers to Your Most Pressing Questions about Memory Loss and Dementia._ Baltimore: Johns Hopkins University Press.

CHAPTER 3

Causes of Dementia

Alzheimer disease is just one type of dementia

C are partners are often surprised to learn that there are more than a hundred different causes of dementia. Working in this field, I am often surprised when someone tells me that their loved one has a specific diagnosis. "My dad has frontotemporal dementia, so his behavior has been particularly challenging to cope with," a woman told me recently. I was sympathetic toward her plight, and I was impressed with her knowledge of the condition. Most care partners do not know the actual cause of a friend or relative's cognitive impairment or how it affects that individual's symptoms and prognosis. I was always pleased when a new resident's paperwork contained detailed information about their mental and physical health, particularly if a professional had made a note that said more about their cognitive status than just "dementia." To best predict a person's symptoms and care needs, it is important to have a complete and accurate diagnosis. There are many different causes of dementia with different characteristics. In this chapter, I discuss the most common forms of dementia.

Is It Dementia?

H ow do you know if someone has dementia? Is there a possibility that their cognitive changes are a result of normal aging, temporary, perhaps caused by delirium, or are instead mild cognitive impairment? Recall from chapter 2 that dementia is the medical term for a *group of symptoms*. For someone to receive a diagnosis of dementia, two or more areas of intellectual ability need to be sufficiently impaired, the symptoms must begin in adulthood, and the person is awake and alert, meaning that they are not drowsy or intoxicated. Although age-related decline in some areas of cognitive functioning is expected, dementia-related decline is significant enough to interfere with a person's daily life. For example, forgetting why you walked into a room is normal, but forgetting how the television remote or telephone works is indicative of a problem (Mace and Rabins, p. 339).

Mild cognitive impairment, or MCI, is a slight but noticeable decline in memory and other cognitive functions. MCI is not dementia, although many people living with MCI do develop some form of dementia over time. Delirium is an acute episode of confusion. It appears suddenly, and it is commonly caused by a urinary tract infection, a fall, a stroke, or an adverse medication interaction. I discuss delirium and MCI in chapter 2.

Alzheimer Disease

Because Alzheimer disease (AD) is the most common cause of dementia, it gets the most attention from researchers and activists. In chapters 1 and 2, I discussed the difference between Alzheimer disease and dementia. To repeat that point: Alzheimer disease is one type of dementia. In this book, I use the term Alzheimer disease rather than Alzheimer's disease. They mean the same thing.

In the early stages of Alzheimer disease, the most common symptom is trouble with short-term memory. Short-term memory loss affects a person's ability to remember information they just heard or recall events that happened recently. Caregivers may be incredulous when they are told their loved one's memory is impaired. "But he remembers everything that happened twenty years ago as if it happened yesterday!" they'll say. Long-term memory, or recall of events that happened in the distant past, tends to stick around even in late stages of AD.

As the disease progresses, major symptoms include increased forgetfulness, trouble with language, mood changes, issues with visual and depth perception, impaired thinking, difficulty understanding logic, and trouble making safe decisions. Like other dementias, as AD progresses, people lose their ability to perform most of the activities of daily living. A person's risk for AD increases with age, although it is most common in women over the age of 65. Women make up 70% of skilled nursing facility residents, according to a report by AARP, and numbers are similar in assisted living and other senior living communities.

Vera was in a moderate stage of Alzheimer disease. She was incredibly pleasant, funny, and talkative. Despite her cognitive loss, Vera retained much of her positive and happy personality. Every so often, though, she would suddenly become stubborn or irritable. The mood would pass quickly, and she would go back to being her joyful self.

Vera didn't realize that her short-term memory was impaired, even though she often asked the same question numerous times during a ten-minute conversation. She was also physically healthy for a woman of 92.

As we drove down the street in our community van, Vera pointed to a water tower near her old house. "My son climbed that tower when he was a little boy," she said, shaking her head. "I walked outside and saw him halfway up there! I yelled at him, 'You come down this instant!' Oh boy, were his father and I angry at him!" She laughed. Vera's long-term memory was still in good shape, but she told us this story another five times before we got back to the community.

Frontotemporal Lobar Dementia

*F*rontotemporal lobar dementia (FTLD) or *frontotemporal degeneration* (FTD) is a group of diseases that affect the frontal and temporal lobes of the brain. These forms of dementia commonly affect younger adults, most often in midlife. Clinicians recognize three common forms of FTD: behavioral, language, and movement forms. Because your *frontal lobe* is the part of your brain that controls decision-making and acts as your "filter," it makes sense that someone living with a frontotemporal impairment will often display behavioral challenges. This filter is what prevents you from speaking out of turn, making risky choices, or telling your boss what you really think of her—all things that are difficult to control living with FTD. In language forms of the disease, people often develop symptoms of aphasia, a speech disorder. They may be unable to find words or understand their meaning, or they may lose their ability to speak at all (Mace and Rabins, p. 344). Although memory loss is the hallmark of Alzheimer disease, people living with any of the forms of FTD will likely also see changes related to mood, judgment, and impulse control, such as sexual disinhibition.

Andrew E. Budson and Neil W. Kowall, in their 2014 book *The Handbook of Alzheimer's Disease and Other Dementias*, note that people living with the behavioral form of FTD experience a set of behavioral changes that can make long-term dementia caregiving uniquely challenging (p. 5). Because it can affect people who are in their forties, fifties, or sixties, care partners often fail to realize that their loved one is experiencing dementia-related symptoms. Sometimes, odd behaviors may even get written off as a midlife crisis because they are so out of character for the individual living with FTD.

FTD language disorders affect a person's ability to speak normally. Words become jumbled, terms become vague (saying "the thing" or "it" instead of being specific), and a person's ability to understand language declines.

In FTD movement disorders, automatic muscle functions become impaired. People living with FTD may experience tremors and spasms or difficulty walking and balancing.

People living with FTD can find dementia care communities difficult environments to live in. Most residents are at least a decade older than a person living with FTD. These older residents listen to music, watch movies, or talk about a past that is unfamiliar to younger people with FTD. Individuals with FTD may not fare well in a dementia care community until they are much more progressed in the disease.

Nicholas was excited that he and his wife, Janice, were getting a new floor in their kitchen. They had just begun talking about the process and needed to save up some money before hiring a contractor. Janice told Nicholas that it would probably be another six months before they had the money to pay for the new floor.

One day Janice came home to find that Nicholas had ripped up the entire kitchen floor—without any warning. He had come home from work, decided it was time, and begun taking apart the floorboards. The couple had to live with this change for months before they could afford to hire someone to fix it.

As a result of this sudden behavioral change, Janice took Nicholas to the doctor, where he was eventually diagnosed with the behavioral form of FTD. His inability to make decisions, process information, and self-monitor had caused him to rip up the floor long before the couple was able to pay for it. He had no sense of why this behavior was bizarre or alarming because the filter part of his brain was not working properly.

———————

Vascular Dementia

A stroke or other blood vessel damage in the brain can lead to various types of *vascular dementia* (VaD). VaD is also called *vascular cognitive impairment* (VCI), to show that it is a group of dementias related to cerebrovascular damage. Cerebrovascular damage is often caused by multiple strokes or inflammation of the blood vessels in the brain. One large stroke can also cause vascular dementia.

Someone living with VaD will usually have trouble with shape discrimination, object perception, and spatial awareness. They will also tend to have difficulties with motor coordination, reflex speed, and speech. Vascular dementia affects the way a person walks, sometimes described as a *gait disturbance*. Although these symptoms are common after a person experiences a stroke, they could be signs of VaD. As with most dementias, a person living with VaD will likely have trouble with memory, especially later in the disease. Vascular dementia some- times exists concurrently with Alzheimer disease, meaning individuals can have both causes of dementia.

Lewy Body Diseases

Lewy body diseases are another common cause of dementia. Named after a doctor, Fritz Heinrich Lewy, Lewy bodies are abnormal deposits of protein that build up inside brain cells. Three different diseases comprise this group.

1. Dementia with Lewy bodies (DLB)
2. Parkinson disease dementia (PDD)
3. Parkinson disease (PD)

Parkinson disease is a type of Lewy body disease, but people living with PD do not always have or develop dementia. You can have Parkinson disease dementia, however, in which dementia symptoms manifest shortly after a PD diagnosis. People who have DLB may have some Parkinsonism symptoms, but they do not have a complete Parkinson diagnosis.

A few symptoms set Lewy body diseases apart from other dementias. People living with a Lewy body disease tend to have a fluctuating degree of impairment. People living with DLB or PDD also tend to hallucinate, often seeing or hearing things like children or animals that are not present. Strange, complex paranoia can accompany these vivid visual hallucinations. Although people living with other dementias can hallucinate, it isn't as common. If you notice that your family member or friend is hallucinating and hasn't experienced hallucinations before, seek medical attention immediately. It could be a sign that something else is wrong, such as a medication reaction or negative interaction between two medications. If they hallucinate regularly, however, do not make the experience of hallucinating even scarier for the person. Instead, make sure to agree with what they are seeing. More information on how to agree with their reality—and why—is in chapter 6.

Other Dementias

Although Alzheimer disease, VaD, DLB, and FTD are the most common forms of dementia, a person living with dementia could receive a different diagnosis or even have several overlapping diagnoses. It's incredibly important that your family member or friend receives a full medical review to determine whether they have dementia. A brain tumor, for example, can cause a potentially reversible type of dementia. Without a thorough examination by a physician, though, the symptoms could be mistaken for Alzheimer disease.

One potential cause of dementia that is gaining more attention is traumatic brain injury (TBI), especially repeated TBI. A TBI is very serious. Common causes of TBI include motor vehicle accidents, falls, violent encounters, sports-related concussions, and combat injuries. The symptoms of a TBI depend on the location of the damage, which explains why people who have a TBI in their frontal lobe have the same symptoms as someone who developed frontotemporal lobar dementia. It has been suggested that brain trauma leads to Alzheimer disease or FTD (Mace and Rabins, p. 348).

People with a history of alcohol abuse are at a greater risk for dementia, due to a vitamin deficiency and a cascade of other factors, such as a history of physical fights or falls. It is possible for someone with alcohol-associated dementia to recover some of their normal functioning—provided that they stop drinking and adopt a healthier lifestyle, including taking vitamin supplements (Mace and Rabins, p. 341).

Depression can be a cause of dementia. Depression can also be the first sign of a person's dementia. Depression affects an individual's memory and other cognitive functioning. Even if the depression does not cause dementia, the depressive disorder must be treated (Mace and Rabins, p. 343).

LATE, or limbic-predominant age-related TDP-43 encephalopathy, is another cause of dementia that scientists are actively researching. It is similar to Alzheimer disease, and researchers hypothesize that some patients have been misdiagnosed, even post-autopsy. Development of LATE tends to happen after the age of 80 and affects predominantly the medial temporal area of the brain, along with the hippocampus, which is critical for learning and memory (Nelson et al.).

Summary

Alzheimer disease isn't the only form of dementia. I have introduced you to several other common and less common dementia diseases. When you think about dementia, recognize that it is more than just a memory problem.

Instead, dementia is group of symptoms caused by many different diseases of cognitive loss. I believe this is why it's so important to say "dementia" instead of "Alzheimer disease and dementia" or just "Alzheimer disease."

Putting It into Practice

Starting the dementia caregiving journey can be an overwhelming experience: Where do you start? What do you need to find out? It may help to write down the answers to these questions so you can begin thinking through that initial diagnosis.

Do you know the cause of your loved one's dementia? What is it?

_____

Even if you do not know the cause, what are some of your loved one's symptoms? What do they often say or ask about?

_____

What do they do when they are happy?

_____

What do they do when they are agitated or anxious?

_____

RESOURCES

AARP Public Policy Institute. 2021. Women and Long-Term Care. https://assets.aarp.org /rgcenter/il/fs77r_ltc.pdf.

Alzheimer's Association. 2021. Is Alzheimer's Genetic? https://www.alz.org/alzheimers -dementia/what-is-alzheimers/causes-and -risk-factors/genetics.

Budson, A. E., and N. W. Kowall. 2014. *The Handbook of Alzheimer's Disease and Other Dementias*. West Sussex: John Wiley & Sons.

Mace, N. L., and P. V. Rabins. 2011. *The 36-Hour Day: A Family Guide to Caring for People Who Have Alzheimer Disease, Related Dementias, and Memory Loss*, 5th ed. Baltimore: Johns Hopkins University Press.

Nelson, P. T., et al. 2019. Limbic-predominant age-related TDP-43 encephalopathy (LATE): consensus working group report. *Brain* awz099: https://doi.org/10.1093/brain /awz099.

CHAPTER 4

Stages of Dementia

Understanding dementia's course

One of the tasks at my first full-time, post-graduate-school dementia care job was to "stage" my residents. Once a month, I would go through my list of residents and assign each of them a number between one and seven based on their level of functioning. A one meant, technically, that the person had "no impairment." None of my residents met this criteria. Seven was "very advanced," and all the other numbers meant something in between. Staging residents was a challenging task for me, and I came to find that this was something I did not enjoy. It was difficult to assign a number to a person's impairment. I knew that it was useful information because it helped us track each resident's decline as the disease progressed. But it was hard. Frankly, each day seemed different: my residents were human beings, not robots. They had good days and bad days, just like we all do. If Mary Ellen was still battling a urinary tract infection, of course her impairment was going to be more significant than it had been before the infection. If Bill had recently come back from the hospital, his impairment could swing from about a three to maybe a six, but with hope for improvement.

Number scales are intended to be clinical, and families of those living with dementia rely on them for information. It can be a daunting task to talk to a care partner about "where on the scale" their loved one falls. In this chapter, we examine different staging tools, identify the signs and symptoms of each stage, and talk about why dementia is a group of terminal diseases.

Different Tools for Staging Dementia

One common staging tool is the Functional Assessment Staging Tool, or FAST, developed by Dr. Barry Reisberg. The FAST scale is based on an individual's functional abilities.

A number one on the scale means that there are no reported or perceived difficulties. There is a distinct difference, however, between numbers two and three. In stage three, early dementia, a person will begin struggling with changing conditions at home and at work. The scale becomes more detailed and layered as the stages progress, with stages six and seven utilizing letters to denote substages of the progressive condition.

The Global Deterioration Scale (GDS), also developed by Dr. Reisberg, is another scale that divides dementia into seven stages. The GDS does not have a letter-number breakdown in later stages of the disease process. Instead, stage seven, "Severe Dementia," is when "All verbal abilities are lost over the course of this stage. Frequently there is no speech at all—only unintelligible utterances and rare emergence of seemingly forgotten words and phrases. Incontinent of urine, requires assistance toileting and feeding. Basic psychomotor skills, e.g., ability to walk, are lost with the progression of this stage. The brain appears to no longer be able to tell the body what to do. Generalized rigidity and developmental neurologic reflexes are frequently present" (Reisberg, p. 7).

The Clinical Dementia Rating (CDR) scale is a five-point scale used to rate a person's memory, orientation, judgment, problem-solving skills, community affairs (that is, level of independence out in the world), home life and hobbies, and personal care needs. This rating is obtained by interviewing both the patient and the patient's caregiver or care partners. Like the FAST scale, the CDR scale takes into account a person's functioning at home, work, and leisure. A copy of the CDR is included in the appendix at the end of this book.

These are a few examples of dementia staging tools. There are numerous other scales and measurement tools out there for staging dementia. It is important that you know what scale your loved one's provider is using when they talk about dementia, because, as you may have realized, hearing that your loved one is a three on the CDR will mean something quite different than hearing that they are a five on the GDS or FAST Scale.

It's not uncommon to hear a professional refer to a person living with dementia as being in "mild/early, moderate/middle, or advanced/late stages" of dementia. While this is not a standardized clinical scale, this shorthand can be helpful when communicating with providers or memory care communities about your loved one. For example, upon calling a new dementia care community, you will probably be asked to share your friend or family member's stage of dementia. Instead of saying "stage five on the FAST scale," you can say "a moderate stage."

People with mild or early-stage dementia often have some issues with their memory and decision-making skills. You may find that you can hold a normal fifteen-minute conversation with a person in an early stage of dementia, but then you begin to notice irregularities in their conversation or behavior over time. Their judgment may seem a little odd, or perhaps they've forgotten about an important appointment. If you are a passenger in a car with them, you may notice that they are losing the ability to safely drive a vehicle.

When you meet someone in a moderate stage of dementia, you will immediately notice their level of cognitive decline. Many people living with moderate stages of dementia are not fully aware of their impairments, however, which may cause their judgment and decision-making to be particularly affected. People living with dementia often remain in a moderate stage for years. During this stage your friend or loved one will experience behavioral changes, such as withdrawal from social activities or moodiness.

Someone in a moderate stage cannot and should not live independently.

A person living with severe or late-stage dementia needs constant physical and psychological care. Previously simple tasks like toileting or feeding themselves now require assistance. The individual requires a great deal of supervision to stay safe. A person with late-stage dementia will continue to decline and will eventually pass away from the disease.

Importance of Staging

Staging is a useful if imperfect tool to help us better understand where someone living with dementia is in the progression of their particular illness. Staging also gives us a common language we can use with one another to talk about the disease. However, people can become overly dependent on the numbers. I once had a woman find me after a conference and tell me, "My husband is in stage four of dementia with Lewy bodies. How long does he have to live?" I was taken aback by this question and didn't know how to answer. She persisted, "Can you give me a general amount of time?" I shook my head. "No," I explained, "because it would be irresponsible of me to take a guess like that. We have no idea what will happen in the future. He could be alive for years, or he could have a terrible fall and pass away in a couple of weeks' time."

The woman was frustrated that I refused to give her an amount of time that her husband had left to live, but I truly believed it would be inappropriate for me

to do so. I thought back to a resident I had, Candice, who was in an early-moderate stage of dementia, probably a five on the FAST scale or a four on the GDS. Candice needed assistance, and by all accounts she would have years left of life. One day, though, she fell, hit her head on the floor, and was hospitalized. Candice passed away within a week of the fall. Although she had been fairly early in her dementia progression, the fall pushed her dementia stage to a seven.

Sometimes dementia progresses slowly for years and then suddenly speeds up. Relatively stable periods are called plateaus because of the flat, generally unchanging progression of the disease (Mace and Rabins, p. 342). Staging is important because it provides information about how the majority of people progress in the disease and some sense of a road map. I always encourage families to remember, however, that the road map is just an approximation. Expect someone living with dementia to take detours on that map, ending up in a very different place than the family anticipated. What often happens is that an individual living with dementia will be going along, barely progressing—at least noticeably—in their disease, and then something will happen. This "something" is called a *precipitating event*, which is an event that causes something else to happen, such as a steep decline. (Precipitating events are explained further in chapter 34.) A precipitating event could be a fall, a bad urinary tract infection, or hospitalization. In Candice's case, the fall was the precipitating event; it caused her to progress suddenly in her dementia. If she hadn't passed away, Candice likely would have gotten a little better (say, from a seven to a six on the FAST scale), but she might never have returned to her original baseline (a five on the FAST scale). After the decline following a precipitating event, families will often ask, "Will my loved one get better?" It is hard to know the answer. Perhaps the best way to answer this question is, "Maybe, but probably not back to where they were before the event occurred."

Why Is Dementia Terminal?

Dementia is the sixth leading cause of death in the United States. What makes dementia a terminal disease? In other words, how does dementia end a person's life? Since dementia affects a person's brain and overall functioning, the simple answer is, if your brain isn't working well, the rest of your body cannot function well, either. The last stages of dementia typically signal that an individual has less than a year of life left, although you may have met individuals—as I have—who live well past their expected timeline.

Let's take Candice as an example to explore the above question. Was it the fall or dementia that caused Candice's death? The answer is both. Dementia primed Candice for a serious fall, and the fall caused further injury that directly caused her death. Candice may not have fallen if her brain had been working properly, telling her body what to do and instructing her muscles to move properly as they had for so many years.

Choking is another common precipitating event. Someone with late-stage dementia might aspirate food while eating because it is difficult for them to chew and swallow their food. Because the dementia has also weakened their immune system and forced them to spend more time lying down because they can no longer walk or get around easily, they are at risk for pneumonia. Sometimes, a person living with dementia will instead begin dying as their brain slowly shuts down. Dementia is made up of a group of terminal diseases, which means that dementia progressively causes damage to the brain tissue until it reaches a point where it begins to turn off life-critical functions. You may hear a health care professional describe this as "their body forgetting how to breathe" or "their brain forgetting to regulate their heartbeat."

Dying with Dementia

Patton was dying, but his daughter was having trouble letting him go. He showed all the signs of what we call "active dying." Active dying is the final days or hours of the dying process. Patton spent all his time in bed, usually with his eyes closed. Occasionally he would open them, but he would close them again without seeming to see or focus on anyone in the room. His daughter insisted that the periods of restlessness were a sign that he was doing better, but they were just something that comes with active dying. She insisted that he not have too much morphine, as she was worried it could kill him. Patton's hospice nurse consoled her. "I promise we are giving him the right amount," she said. "He is dying, and we want to ensure that he's comfortable as he passes."

In the weeks prior to someone's passing, they often sleep more, withdrawal socially, lose interest in eating or drinking, and become restless. I recall one resident who in the weeks before he passed constantly asked our staff to move him in his wheelchair to another part of the hallway. "I think I have to go somewhere, but I don't know where that is," he offered to me one day. I thought of that quote a couple days after he died and found myself wondering if he'd known that he was dying—that he knew he needed to "go somewhere."

In the days and hours prior to death, the individual will have decreased response to stimuli and unfocused vision. Their breathing will change, including the beginnings of congestion or what is called a "death rattle." A death rattle sounds like a low gurgling sort of sound, which can be stressful for some family members to hear. Often, there is shortness of breath. The person will have low blood pressure and cold, mottled skin. Mottling is a bluish-purple tone that moves over the skin on the extremities of a dying individual. The person may experience a surge of energy, almost as if they are recovering suddenly, only to decline again later (Kenny, pp. 179–88).

Understanding Death and Dying

Understanding and accepting death and the dying process can be challenging for loved ones of the individual who is passing away. I recommend Dr. Anne Kenny's book *Making Tough Decisions about End-of-Life Care in Dementia*, also published by Johns Hopkins University Press. She covers planning for advance directives and decision-making processes at the end of life, wills, guardianships, conversations to discuss with attorneys; explains the stages of death and dying; and discusses the grieving process. Her information is immensely helpful, even if the later stages of the disease seem far away.

In the next section, we review how families can continue to enjoy time and experiences with their loved ones living with dementia. It's not all doom and gloom. There are so many beautiful moments that occur as someone moves through their dementia journey.

Putting It into Practice

I caution against making your own dementia diagnosis using the information in this chapter. That said, I believe the scales can be helpful for providing additional information or encouraging you to speak to a physician for further answers.

Do you know your loved one's stage of dementia?

_____

Which scale is used by your loved one's health care partner to assess dementia?

_____

Which dementia staging tool does the memory care community use?

_____

RESOURCES

Five Wishes. 2021. Advance Directive. https:// fivewishes.org/Home.

Kenny, A. 2018. *Making Tough Decisions about End-of-Life Care in Dementia*. Baltimore: Johns Hopkins University Press.

Mace, N. L., and P. V. Rabins. 2011. *The 36-Hour Day: A Family Guide to Caring for People Who Have Alzheimer Disease, Related Dementias,* *and Memory Loss*, 5th ed. Baltimore: Johns Hopkins University Press.

Reisberg, B. 1983. The Global Deterioration Scale for Assessment of Primary Degenerative Dementia. https://www.fhca.org /members/qi/clinadmin/global.pdf.

Washington University in St Louis. 2001. CDR Scoring Table. https://knightadrc.wustl.edu /cdr/PDFs/CDR_Table.pdf.

CHAPTER 5

Medications

Kelly was the most anxious resident I ever had. I have always prided myself on being able to create a calming atmosphere for my residents and to refocus them on a new activity during their bouts of fear or anxiety, but Kelly tested every one of my skills. If I could measure Kelly's anxiety on a scale from one to ten, ten being the highest, I would say that Kelly operated regularly at about an eight—and that was normal. When she hit ten, Kelly was completely inconsolable. At an eight, Kelly regularly forgot new information. At a ten, her ability to remember things she heard one minute ago evaporated: she could not hear or pay attention to what care partners said to her. Kelly's daughter came to visit almost every day, and telling Kelly that her daughter was on the way calmed her down for about ten seconds. "I want to see my daughter!" she'd cry, tears spilling out of her eyes as she darted up and down the hallway, looking for anyone to ask about the upcoming visit.

It was heartbreaking and exhausting to watch, so I can only imagine how difficult it was to actually be inside Kelly's mind while all that anxiety was ripping her apart. I insisted to my boss—who worked on another floor—that we desperately needed medication to decrease Kelly's anxiety. "We don't want to use medication as a first resort," she said. "Trust me," I sighed, "this is far from the first resort." We had tried just about everything: sensory rooms, baby dolls, stuffed animals, games and crafts, snacks, music, staff attention and hand-holding, midday naps, and more.

As an anxious person myself, I was committed to finding a solution for Kelly. I know what it feels like to be worked up and unable to relax, and I cannot imagine what it must feel like when you are also living with dementia. After much back-and-forth with the attending psychiatric nurse and Kelly's family, we tried a medication that finally helped decrease some of her anxiety. Although it didn't eliminate the anxiety, the medication helped Kelly feel a bit more grounded and made it easier for us to calm her down.

Using Medication in Dementia Care

The use of medication in dementia caregiving is tricky, to say the least. Many physicians are hesitant to prescribe certain medications for older adults, but it is of particular concern for those living with dementia. In Kelly's case, her nurse put her on a medication called a neuroleptic (or antipsychotic). Neuroleptics are well known for their potentially dangerous side effects, particularly among older populations. Many of these drugs have a black box warning printed on the label that tells the user and the user's physician the *contraindications* of taking the medication. For example, a medication may increase the risk of falls, infection, or stroke in someone with a dementia diagnosis, so it may be contraindicated for someone living with dementia. In Kelly's extreme situation, however, a neuroleptic was the best course of action. Her particular medication did not need to be taken every day, and so it was prescribed PRN, meaning "as needed."

In this chapter, I talk about medications for the treatment of both symptoms of dementia, such as memory loss and confusion, and symptoms of anxiety and depression. With any discussion of medications, it's important to consult with your loved one's health care provider about medications, including what the drug is being prescribed for, what are the potential side effects, and whether the drug can interact with other medications.

As I say often, medications exist for a reason, but they are not the sole solution to a problem. I always recommend trying to solve a problem with environmental changes before trying medication. If the problem is persistent enough to warrant more attention—in Kelly's case, for example—it may be worth it to try combining medication with environmental changes. We found that after providing Kelly medication, we were better able to engage her in an activity.

It is worth repeating: never use medications unless absolutely necessary. For example, a community that is unlocked and constantly has residents walking out the door should not begin medicating the residents who try to leave. Instead, the residents who cannot be redirected may fair better in a secured dementia care community. It's not appropriate or legal to restrict a person because they are engaging in a normal activity such as seeking the exits. "Snowing someone" means that you load them up with medication so that they become sleepy and almost nonresponsive. This is gross misconduct and completely avoidable in most scenarios. In chapter 12, I talk about using your dementia detective skills. Use these skills first whenever you encounter a problem in someone's behavior. In addition, ask yourself if what you are noticing is fixable without the introduction of new medications.

You will meet some professionals who say, "Never use medication in dementia care" and others who say, "Medication is absolutely necessary and should always be an option." If you have a loved one who is reeling from anxiety and fearfulness, you will probably err on the side of "medication should be an option." If you or another relative don't believe in using medication, that's okay, but recognize that it's about what the person living with dementia needs to live a balanced life.

Understanding the Basics of Medications

Many older adults, even ones with dementia, are taking numerous medications at the same time. When an older person is seeing two, three, or even more physicians, this may be part of the reason that they end up with so many prescriptions. One of the things that I like best about places like Penn Medicine's Penn Memory Center and the University of Pittsburgh's Alzheimer Disease Research Center is that they review all of a patient's prescribed and over-the-counter medications. Patients are asked to bring in all of their medications so that the attending professionals can review what they are taking. Perhaps some combinations of the medications are contraindicated, or maybe one of the pills could be causing side effects that mimic symptoms of dementia. Before making a dementia diagnosis, it's important to rule out side effects from things like medications.

Keep track of what your loved one living with dementia is taking. Medication management is incredibly challenging for someone living with dementia, and relying on them to manage their daily meds may not be the best plan. I have watched families struggle with calendars, pill reminder systems, apps, and electronic talking medication aids to allow their loved one living with dementia to continue managing their own medications. My advice to these families is: *stop*. There's a much greater chance that the person living with the disease will forget what they've already taken and take another, or completely forget to take an important pill. Don't challenge them with reminders or ask, "Did you take your medication today?" because you probably won't get an accurate answer. I have frequently heard the statement, "We knew something was wrong with her when she stopped taking her medication properly."

Side Effects and Individual Differences

Understand that the same medication can have very different side effects—and effects in general—on two different people. This is one of the main reasons you should never share your prescribed medication with someone else. You just don't know how their body will handle it. Our bodies also process medication differently as we age, which is why some medications will be prescribed in lower doses for older adults than for younger people. Many medications require a "stepping down" period before someone completely ceases taking a pill. I had a man ask me at a workshop recently, "Can I take my wife off her medication? The nursing home where she lives insists she needs it, but I think they just don't know how to redirect her properly." I explained to him that although this may be true, and that perhaps she didn't need it, it was not entirely up to him whether she took her pills. I suggested that he consult with her physician and express his feelings about the neuroleptic she'd been prescribed and was taking almost daily. Storming in and demanding that the community she lived in stop giving it to her would do nothing. The nursing staff was working off a doctor's orders, and stopping a medication suddenly can be dangerous.

Current Medications

What medications are available for someone living with dementia? Do any medications stop or prevent the decline from a particular cause of dementia? Sadly, there are currently no medications that stop or prevent the decline associated with dementia. There are, however, medications that treat the *symptoms* of dementia, for example, helping someone with short-term memory loss. An individual may see positive effects after taking their daily pills. But once the medication wears off, the underlying problem is still there. Common medications for dementia include Razadyne, Aricept, Exelon, and Namenda. Do these medications actually work? According to Peter V. Rabins in the book *Is It Alzheimer's?*, "The evidence is clear that these medications work better than a sugar pill, but there is disagreement among experts about how much of a benefit they provide, how long they should be prescribed, whether they should be prescribed in very high dosages, and whether they are worth the cost" (p. 46).

You may be thinking, "Is there a point to taking any of these medications, then?" Currently, most physicians say yes. Researchers have found that patients on these medications have about a six-month window of improvement in thinking and daily function when treated with Aricept, Razadyne, or Exelon. In *Is It Alzheimer's?* Dr. Rabins writes, "About one-third of people with Alzheimer disease and Parkinson disease dementia experience a measurable improvement in thinking and daily function when treated with the anti-cholinesterase medications Razadyne (galantamine), Exelon (rivastigmine), or Aricept (donepezil)." Namenda acts as an NMDA (N-methyl-D-aspartate) receptor antagonist, which in layman's terms means that it is a slightly different medication than the other three. When it's prescribed alone, it's not as effective at treating AD as the other medications, but it is often combined with the use of

Aricept, Razadyne, or Exelon for a more effective concoction.

Six months is not a long window of improvement, and I have met countless people living with dementia who have been on Aricept for years. Why have they stayed on a medication when its effectiveness window is, by most accounts, so short? The reason is that many physicians are reluctant to take a patient off a drug that *could* be having a positive effect or, in the very least, preventing a more negative effect.

In essence, getting a person on or off medication is a decision that needs to be made by the primary care partners and the medical professionals they work with. In the activity at the end of the chapter, I've included a short medication tracker for you to use. Look at all the medications that your loved one is taking. What are they for? How often do they need to be taken? I always recommend bringing the entire collection to a doctor's office during a checkup. It's a good idea to review a person's medication list regularly.

Ongoing Research

I regularly read new studies about ongoing research in the fight against dementia. Most of this research centers around finding the cause of certain forms of dementia, so that the researchers can search for medications to treat it. The problem that researchers currently face is that we don't know what causes many of the different forms of dementia. It can therefore be challenging to find something that treats the thing that is responsible for the disease rather than treating the symptoms of the disease.

Until recently, most researchers were focused on what is called the "amyloid hypothesis," which proposes that a buildup of beta-amyloid protein is the main cause of Alzheimer disease. This breakdown could be the cause of cognitive and motor problems, but we don't know that for sure. New research shows that cognitive decline appears to be happening prior to the buildup of beta-amyloid in the brain.

There is hope. Researchers are looking into other potential causes of dementia, the impact of heredity, germ theories, and even the use of insulin as medication for dementia. There is also a great deal of research into diet and how it can affect a person's risk for dementia. Recognize, though, that while a heart-healthy diet has been shown to have some preventative impact in dementia, it is not a cure-all. And switching a person living with dementia to a challenging, restrictive diet will prove more harmful than good. Most people living with dementia, particularly in later stages, prefer sweeter foods.

You may be thinking, "Why do I hear about dementia all the time?" For one, if you're reading this book, you are probably providing care to someone with dementia. Your Internet search history influences the ads and articles that pop up in your web feed every day. The people you spend time with know you have a loved one with dementia and talk with you about it. And as a society, we are talking about dementia more than ever. Until recently, it was not uncommon to hear someone say, "Oh, grandma is getting a little senile!" These days, that's a red flag for most families because they know that "senile" is code for dementia, and that perhaps we can do something to help grandma's cognition. Over the years that I've been working in this field, I've seen a shift for the better in how we approach dementia care.

Putting It into Practice

Medication Tracker

What medications are being taken by my loved one living with dementia? List names, doses, and requirements for taking them.

Name of Medication	Strength and Frequency	Condition Medication Taken for	Physician Who Prescribed Medication	Notes

What is each medication for? Educate yourself on what these medications do. Ask your loved one's physician about the purpose of each medication.

Do any of these medications have a black box warning?

_____

When is the last time a health care professional reviewed all these medications?

_____

What about supplements—including teas, vaping products, and other items—that your loved one may use? Be specific.

_____

RESOURCES

Alzheimer's Association. 2021. Medications for
    Memory, Cognition, and Dementia-Related
    Behaviors. https://www.alz.org/alzheimers
    -dementia/treatments/medications-for
    -memory.
Rabins, P. V. 2020. *Is It Alzheimer's? 101 Answers
    to Your Most Pressing Questions about
    Memory Loss and Dementia.* Baltimore: Johns
    Hopkins University Press.

PART II

Communicating with People Living with Dementia

Before we can discuss details about memory care communities, we need to talk about communication in dementia caregiving. If we don't know how to communicate with someone living with dementia, we can't possibly consider the healthiest, safest way to transition them to a care community. In this section I tackle many of the myths that we hear about dementia care, such as "A person with dementia will forget their family members." I introduce my proven communication strategy, Embracing Their Reality, and tell you how and why it works far better than simply "redirecting, distracting, or validating a person living with dementia.

CHAPTER 6

Embracing Someone's Reality

How to use positive dementia care communication

Embracing Their Reality

When caring for someone living with dementia, you may come to realize that their perception of reality is not the same as yours. They may tell you things that are not true and things that seem to you completely impossible. Care partners have often confided in me that they "feel as though they're lying" if they "go along with" what their loved one is saying. "I don't know," an adult daughter will offer, "when Mom talks about Dad still being alive, I just feel like I have to correct her! He died years ago . . . it's not fair to her that she doesn't know the truth!"

When I first started working in dementia care environments, I learned the basics of positive dementia communication from experts that had come before me. Three of the main concepts that I learned were *redirection, distraction, and validation.* I was taught that when someone living with dementia asks you about something that is not true, your goal should be to redirect the conversation or distract them from it entirely. For example, if a person with dementia asked,

"Where is my mother?" you might say, "Sounds like you really miss your mom!" This would be validation: you're accepting what she's saying, but you aren't going much further than that. A redirection or a distraction would be to accept what they said and then change the subject, or focus on a new task, such as, "I don't know where she is. Let's go work on this puzzle together." I also learned that you should never lie to someone living with dementia. This comes from Naomi Feil's Validation Therapy. Feil asserts that it is cruel to lie and suggests that it may confuse the person further.

Although these concepts were great building blocks for my professional development and may be techniques that work in certain circumstances, I found that redirection, distraction, and validation didn't work in all situations. For example, I was once asked by one of my residents where her husband was. Using what I had learned, I replied, "Sounds like you miss your husband." The resident shook her head, annoyed. "Of course, but where is he? Why does no one answer my questions!" she sighed, exasperated. I was a bit shocked to realize that my training hadn't fully prepared me for real conversations with adults living with dementia. That was when I began working on my own concept: Embracing Their Reality™. When you embrace someone's reality, you recognize that their worldview has shifted, and that it's your job to shift with it. It is never our place to correct someone living with dementia, and feeling like we're "lying" to them only makes us worry that we're doing the wrong thing. Instead, we need to join the individual in their new reality; if it's true for them, it's true for us. In fact, it would be cruel and likely confusing to tell them the truth of our reality. How can you do this effectively? We will cover this later in the chapter.

Embracing someone's reality may make you feel as though you're lying. *But it's not about lying, it's about being truthful according to their reality.* Even if what they are saying is not true for us, it is still true for them. Although Feil asserts that it's "lying" if you engage in their past reality, I argue that the opposite is true: telling that person what is true in your reality but is no longer true in theirs is the lie. What I'm suggesting you do is find out what is true for them, and then go along with that. I believe that saying, "It sounds like you miss your mom," distracting from the subject, ignoring it, or trying to move on too quickly past the conversation results in the person living with dementia never feeling heard or understood. When we avoid fully Embracing Their Reality, we do the person living with dementia a disservice.

I once overheard a nurse arguing with a man who was living with dementia. He was irate and banging on the door to another resident's room. "That's my wife!" he yelled. "My wife is in there, and you better let me in to see her!"

"That is not your wife. Your wife doesn't live here," the nurse said. "You cannot come in here while we are getting this woman changed." The more she told him this, the more frustrated and angry he became.

"That is my wife. That's my wife. Let me in there! You think I don't know what my wife looks like?" he shouted, slamming his walker into the door. This resident wasn't his wife, but telling him this wasn't helping the situation.

I walked up and laid my hand on his shoulder. "Hey, let's wait out here for your wife. She'll be ready soon," I assured him. He calmed down immediately and sat with me. After talking with him for a couple minutes, I went back to find the nurse and suggested she avoid arguing with him. She became defensive and said she did not want to lie.

"It's not lying," I explained. "If he believes that she's his wife, that's what is true for him. Let him think that she's his wife, avoid arguing with him, and I'll keep him company out here while we wait."

———————

The nurse's response was, unfortunately, a typical one. Care partners want to do the "right" thing—especially when caring for a parent or spouse—and telling the person the truth of our reality often seems like the right thing. Many caregivers ask me, "Is lying really the best option?" They have spent their whole lives being truthful with their loved ones, so why should they stop now?

When Embracing Someone's Reality
Is Challenging

This technique takes practice. I often see some puzzled looks from the crowd when I first begin teaching Embracing Their Reality in workshops and seminars, and I always emphasize that it takes practice. No one is good at this overnight, especially because it's counterintuitive to most of what we understand about treating disease. When a person has cancer, for example, we speak with them about treatment options, listen to their fears and concerns, voice our own fears and concerns, and consult further with physicians. Dementia caregiving is different.

One woman I worked with had to take multiple medications. Each day when I went to check on her, she was convinced that she had already taken her heart medication. "I already took that today," she would tell me. "I took it at six o'clock this morning, and no one was here to see me take it. But I remember taking it, and I am not taking another one."

The pills were still in her pillbox, so she had clearly not taken anything. But she truly believed she had already taken the pills and refused to take them "again," which made sense in her reality.

"I just called your doctor, and he would like you to take a second dose," I explained, thinking quickly.

"Oh, okay, thank you for calling him!" She smiled, holding out her hand for the pills. This made sense in her reality, and she accepted the first of her medications for the day.

———

Keep in mind that the reality and the timeline of a person with dementia are not always the same as yours. It's also imperative to remember that finding the right solution takes time, listening, and sometimes a few creative questions. It may take a few tries before you figure out how to embrace their reality in that moment. Once caregivers understand this, life can be less complicated and less hurtful for all involved.

Bella did not want to get off the bus. She had arrived back at our dementia care community after a doctor's appointment, and she didn't understand where she was. "This isn't my house," she said, her voice rising. "I want this bus to take me to my house, where it picked me up!" No matter what I said, Bella remained determined to sit on this bus forever.

"I am not getting off this bus," she argued. "You are trying to trick me. This is not my house, and I want this bus to take me to my house right this instant." Of course, she had not lived at home for years, and we needed to get her off the vehicle. She was far enough into dementia that she was confused about her location but aware enough to argue vehemently that she did not wish to get off the bus.

I had to embrace her reality and understand her situation. I explained that we would need to get on another bus because this bus only took a certain route. She insisted that we move to the next stop. I convinced the bus driver to drive us around for ten minutes and then park behind the building.

"Okay, we're here!" I said with some enthusiasm when we arrived back at the community. She was not pleased, but I promised that we would only be staying at this "hotel" for a short time. Finally, I was able to coax her off the bus.

———————

I tried multiple tactics to get Bella to follow me off that bus. Eventually, one (or perhaps a combination of techniques) worked. If I had employed only redirection or distraction techniques, they wouldn't have worked. And if I'd stuck to validation therapy, which says "never to lie," I wouldn't have gotten her off the bus, either.

It took me a while to truly understand and define what it meant to embrace someone else's reality: *It was about joining them in their world, wherever that world was.* Even if that world made zero sense to me, it made sense to them. I discovered, too, that it was much more about solving an emotional problem instead of a factual or physical one. Dealing with the emotional issue, not the issue of whether it was true in our reality, was the real solution. For Bella, the issue was not actually whether the bus would take her home, but that she was scared and anxious. By listening to her, I was able to find a way to acknowledge and comfort her fears, and then bring her to a safe place.

The Three Questions

Under normal circumstances, we do not want to ask a lot of questions of someone who is confused. Asking what they did that day, what they ate for breakfast, or what they are planning on doing later all rely on short-term memory, so we don't want to quiz someone for these answers. When we are seeking to understand someone's reality, however, asking three questions can help us better understand our loved one who is living with dementia.

- *Where do you think they are?* You can ask this question when your loved one asks you a direct question, such as "Where's my father?" Instead of providing your own answer, find out where they think their father is. "Where do you think he is?" you should ask. When they tell you the answer, agree with whatever it is, saying something like "Yes, that sounds about right, he's probably at the gym." Then, when you are asked again later, you can just repeat the answer they originally gave you: "I think you told me that he's at the gym." This prevents you from having to make up an answer or potentially say the wrong thing. People usually like the answer that they gave you! Here's another tip: if the person they're asking about is a shared loved one, you can say, "I haven't talked to them in a while." For example, if your mother asks about your brother, who is deceased, "Where's your brother?" you can say, "Hmm, I haven't spoken to him in a while." Your mother may reply, "Huh, me neither," or, "Wait, did he pass away?" You are able to reply, "Yes, but I feel like I talk to him all the time in my head," or, "I pray for him often—I need to do that again tonight."

- *What do you think about this?* This is a question we will explore more fully in chapter 27, where we discuss activities for people with dementia. For now, recognize that this question relates to introducing a baby doll or stuffed animal to someone living with dementia. The goal is to ask them what they think of it, instead of assuming the answer for ourselves. Again, we are going to agree with whatever they say.
- *Can you help me?* This is another question that we are going to delve into in chapter 27. When we ask someone if they can help us, we are telling them that they are important and useful. If we ask someone living with dementia "Can you help me?" instead of asking if they "want" to do something or "want" to help us, then we are engaging them in whatever task we are doing. When we give instructions instead of asking for help, or when we ask, "Do you want to . . . ?" we're not stepping into their shoes and meeting them where they are. By asking "Can you help me?" we're Embracing Their Reality by living in their world, finding out what they need, and then making them feel necessary and helpful.

These three questions help us to better understand someone's reality and then join that reality. As I often ask caregivers, *If we don't know where someone's reality is, how can we go there?*

Putting It into Practice

Let's draw it out. What does your loved one's reality look like? Where is the line between what they believe to be true and what you believe to be true? We may not know for certain exactly how old someone believes they are, but we can probably use some context clues to take an educated guess. Below are some questions to keep in mind as you explore their reality with them.

Note: Remember not to quiz your loved one, but instead seek the answers to these questions through conversation and time spent together.

1. How old does your loved one think they are, approximately?

2. Where does your loved one believe home is?

_____

3. Is there anyone they believe is still alive but has passed away?

_____

4. Are there any traumas or successes in their life they are reliving? For example, I have known veterans who believe that they are still living in war zones.

_____

5. Does your loved one believe they are still working?

_____

6. Do they think they can still safely drive or make health care choices for themselves?

_____

7. Does your loved one have moments where they are more lucid or less confused about what is true for them?

_____

Reflect on what you just recorded. Are the answers significantly different from the answers that are true for you? If so, we can safely assume that your loved one's reality has changed. I want to mention, too, that this is not a bad thing! Often, the reality of a person living with dementia is happier than the reality that we are actually living in: people who have died are still alive, they love their career, or they are still living at home with their parents. Even when their reality isn't happy all the time, it is crucial for us to know where that reality is. It's much easier for us to join their reality when we know how to get there.

RESOURCES

Feil, N. Validation Therapy. *Geriatric Nursing* 13, no. 3 (1992): 129–33. https://doi.org/10.1016/S0197-4572(07)81021-4.

Feil, N., and R. Altman. The Myth of the Therapeutic Lie. 2019. https://vfvalidation.org/wp-content/uploads/2019/05/The-Myth-of-the-Therapeutic-Lie.pdf.

Wonderlin, R. 2021. Dementia by Day (*blog*). https://rachaelwonderlin.com/dementiabyday/dementia-by-day-blog/.

CHAPTER 7

Why Logic, Quizzing, and Reorientation Don't Work

What to do instead

Occasionally, I've had care partners assert that reminding a loved one living with dementia does, in fact, work. "If I just tell her that her mom died years ago, she remembers!" I have had others tell me that they take their mother to the cemetery to prove to her that her husband died years earlier. When I hear these tales of reality orientation, I cringe, for there is nothing worse than reminding someone they should be mourning a loss when perhaps, just for a bit, they've forgotten to feel sad.

Insisting that someone living with dementia share the truth of our reality does not work, at least not for long. What usually happens is the person receiving the bad news will feel sad, then forget the information they learned, but continue to feel sad without knowing why they feel that way. We never want to use logic, quizzing, or reality reorientation to make someone living with dementia "come back" to the reality in which we live.

Reorientation

In dementia care, there are three caregiving techniques to avoid: reorienting, using logic, and giving reminders. The terms *orienting* and *reorienting* refer to a process in which a caregiver brings (or attempts to bring) the person living with dementia into the caregiver's reality. This is the opposite of

Embracing Their Reality and has no place in positive dementia care. Statements like "Your parents have been dead for years" or "You're retired, don't worry about going to work anymore" are examples of reorientation. Both statements are meant to "correct" a person living with dementia, but this approach is unkind and can induce pain. Although it's imperative that we know how to embrace someone's reality, it's also important to know what happens when we do the opposite.

Often, the person living with dementia lives in a much happier reality than the one we inhabit. In their world, their parents are alive or they are looking forward to going to work. Reorienting a person with dementia can be a heartbreaking experience for both parties. It is not only improper care—it's also cruel.

Eva sat in the front room of the community, staring hard out the door. It was still early in the morning, so I was surprised to see her there. Although Eva often sat near the door waiting to "go home," she usually did not feel anxious about it until later in the day. As I walked in the door, I approached her chair. "Hey Eva," I said. "What are you doing here?"

"I just found out that my parents died," Eva explained slowly, tears in her eyes. "One of the girls here just came up and told me that. I cannot believe I missed the funeral. I never got to say goodbye to them." She was heartbroken.

"That's awful!" I said, taking her hand. "But I just found out that their funeral is on Thursday, so you haven't missed it," I offered. I knew full well the funeral wasn't on Thursday, but I picked a day far enough in the future that she'd probably forget I had mentioned it at all. I also wanted to reassure her that she would be able to get there, which was her main concern.

Eva looked up at me with her blue eyes glittering. "I haven't missed it?" she asked.

"No," I said. "And I'll make sure we get you there."

Had I handled that situation differently, such as suggesting that Eva's parents had been dead for years, so she shouldn't worry about the funeral, chaos would probably have ensued. By embracing her reality, I was able to give her closure in her parents' death. Reminding her that they had died years before would not have provided closure at all. In fact, it would have just brought her pain.

Recognize that there are degrees of reorientation. For example, I have had people say to me, "Well, I know not to take her to the cemetery, but when she asks about Dad, I remind her that he passed away." Taking someone to the cemetery is an extreme version of reorientation, but telling a person that a loved one has died is also reorienting them to our reality. Any type of reorientation should be avoided in positive dementia care communication.

Logic

Logic is what we use when we are arguing with someone. We present facts, they present facts, and then we hope that logic will prevail, in that whoever has presented the better facts will "win." This is not the case in dementia communication. We can present as many facts as we want, but it won't solve the problem. When someone living with dementia lives in a different reality than we do, their facts are different than ours. Using our facts to contradict their facts is an exercise in futility. Your frustrated exclamation, "But you haven't showered in a week!" will probably only result in them saying, "Yes I did! I showered yesterday before you came over." That's a tough case to disprove. The answer to the question, "But how do I prove to my friend living with dementia that . . . ?" is "You don't prove anything."

When we remind people living with dementia of facts they do not remember, we remind them that they are living with dementia. We remind them that something is wrong with the way that they think. For example, your mother may not recall that she attended her sister's funeral six years earlier. When she asks where her sister is, it's important that you don't bombard her with *your* truth. By letting her know that her sister is deceased, you are introducing new information into the conversation. In her current reality, your mother is unaware that her sister is deceased, and you just told her, seemingly for the first time. She will no doubt be upset, agitated, and confused. "What else don't I know about?" she may ask herself.

It can be tempting to use logic when dealing with accusations from people living with dementia. It's common for people living with dementia to say things like "Someone is stealing from me" or "My spouse is cheating on me," even when you know that neither of these things is happening. Accusations come down to control: the person feels as though they've lost control of various things happening in their life, and blaming others for losses is much easier than blaming themselves. For example, it is far easier to believe that a nurse has stolen all of your socks than for you to admit you put the socks somewhere and forgot where you placed them. While it's tempting to say, "Why would anyone steal your socks?" it's much easier to say something like, "Wow, I don't think anyone would steal from you, but let me look into it for you." You're not denying their reality, and you're offering to "help" resolve the situation.

We may also believe that a person living with dementia will not remember what we tell them, which can make it tempting to reorient them, if only for a moment. It is important to remember that although a person living with dementia may not remember what they have heard, they can remain confused and upset long after the conversation ends. Emotion has an incredibly strong influence on memory. It is a much simpler—and often happier—approach to just live in that person's reality.

Quizzing

It can be challenging to find things to talk about with people who have short-term memory problems and confusion. We all ask our friends questions like "What have you been up to today?" or "Where did you go to dinner last night?" Carrying on this type of conversation is often difficult for people living with dementia, however. Although they can usually talk about their childhood with ease, recalling recently learned information is nearly impossible. This is why quizzing, or asking numerous questions, is not the preferred way to communicate with a person who is living with dementia.

Eleanor's grandchildren, now adults in their twenties, were excited to see their grandmother. They did not, however, know how to navigate Eleanor's Alzheimer disease. Every time they visited her, they quizzed her about what she had done that day, what she had eaten, and whom she had talked to. They were not trying to be unkind— they just weren't sure what to talk about with their grandmother.

"Hi!" one of the young women greeted Eleanor. "Do you remember who I am?"

Eleanor paused, smiling anxiously. "Well, of course! You're . . . you are . . . um . . ." She stumbled over her words, trying to search her brain for the right information.

"I'm Suzanne, your granddaughter!" the woman said, smiling and attempting to be helpful.

"Of course! Yes, Suzanne, I'm sorry. I'm just having such a busy day. You know how those things are," Eleanor offered, trying to understand why she was struggling to recall her own granddaughter's name and face.

If you have a family member or friend living with dementia, particularly if that person lives in a dementia care community, you may find it tempting to ask her about what she did that day before you arrived. Outside of dementia care, this is normal practice. In dementia care, however, it's not wise to quiz a person about her day. You may receive incorrect information or maybe no information at all.

For example, asking your mother if she went out for ice cream with the rest of the residents when you know that she did is a poor choice. You already know the answer, and asking if she remembers puts her in a compromising position. She may not recall going on an outing, even if it ended only an hour ago. She may also become upset or frustrated if she felt as though she missed out. Along the same lines, asking your mother if she had lunch is also not wise—especially if you already know the answer. Many people living with dementia do not recall short-term memories, particularly those not attached to emotion. Even if she had fun on the ice cream outing or enjoyed a nice lunch, she may have difficulty figuring out when events happened, especially if they are recurring events, like eating lunch. Your mother could be thinking of yesterday's lunch, or even last week's lunch. "No, I didn't eat at all today," she may respond.

As always, it is imperative that you embrace your loved one's reality, whatever that reality is. It is okay to ask about their day, but do not expect a perfect answer. Going along with the story will make the experience positive for everyone.

"What have you been up to today?" Terry's guests asked him.

"Oh boy, we went for a lovely bike ride through the countryside!" Terry exclaimed. "It was so beautiful. We all had such a lovely time."

Terry's guests were clearly puzzled, but they went along with his story. "Wow, that sounds . . . that sounds fun," one offered, clearly confused.

Although Terry had gone on no such bike ride, he believed that he had. In his world, what he had done that morning was completely different than what he had actually been doing. Terry wasn't lying. Because of his dementia, Terry's brain had created a different story that made sense to him. He truly believed he had gone on a bike ride. Perhaps he enjoyed riding bikes in the morning and had done so often as a young adult. Fortunately, because Terry's guests were not quite sure what to make of his story, they decided not to argue.

"Maybe you'll be able to come along next time!" Terry happily told his guests.

Terry's guests did not get an actual answer about what he had done that day. They did, however, hear a colorful story that had played out in Terry's mind. The situation ended positively because Terry's guests agreed with his story. It is important to agree with a person who is living with dementia, even if the story they are telling is a fantasy.

The best way to approach a person living with dementia, especially if you aren't sure they will remember you, is to be calm, positive, and greet them by their preferred name. "Hi, Joan, how are you feeling today?" you may ask. This lets Joan know that you are speaking to her and not to someone else in the room. It also gives her a sense that you are interested in her, and she will be more likely to engage positively with you. It is not uncommon to hear people with dementia say, "How did you know my name!" to a family or staff member at a dementia care community. People are always happy to be addressed personally, and they feel good that someone knows them.

Here's the main takeaway. Reminding your father living with dementia that his parents are dead, that he lives in a skilled nursing facility, or that it is no longer the decade that he thinks it is can be heartbreaking. Your dad may seem to recall this information after you have provided it, but he'll be upset that he forgot it in the first place. After a little while, the facts will leave his mind again. You succeeded in reminding him of the truth, but his foul mood will stick around much longer than the information did. It is a zero-sum game; neither you nor your dad have gained anything in this exchange. A gentle reminder about where the spoons go or what you're eating for dinner is okay. But a reminder about who has passed away and when is not a good idea.

Putting It into Practice

For the following scenarios, provide a response that doesn't rely upon logic, quizzing, or reorientation.

Your loved one tells you:
"The nurse's aide took my favorite bracelet, the one with the blue stones, and won't give it back! I'm tired of people taking my things!"

How can you respond?

_____

Your loved one tells you:
"I don't need a shower because I already took one this morning!"

How can you respond?

_____

Your loved one tells you:
"I just found out that my brother died, and someone told me I'm missing the service because I can't leave here."

How can you respond?

_____

RESOURCES

Gerteis, M., S. Edgman-Levitan, J. Daley, et al.
    (eds). 1993. *Through the Client's Eyes:*
    Understanding and Promoting Client-Centered
    Care. San Francisco: Jossey-Bass.
National Institute on Aging. 2017. Tips for
    Communicating with a Confused Patient.
    https://www.nia.nih.gov/health/tips
    -communicating-confused-patient.

CHAPTER 8

Yes, and...
Improvisation and Dementia

Applying improvisation techniques from the theatre to dementia care

Improvisational comedy is an art form that combines acting techniques, humor, mental quickness, and teamwork to create a unique performance piece. More simply, improv is when teams of two to eight people get onstage and make up a play in front of an audience. Usually what happens is the performers get a suggestion of a word or theme from the audience, then take that suggestion and turn it into a performance. Two people step out onto the stage and start a scene together with no preparation for what is going to happen within that scene. It seems out of the ordinary to newcomers. How do they know what to do? Improv is all about listening and building upon what has already been said or done. The performers find related characters, topics, and words to form scenes that flow together.

If you've ever watched the popular television show *Whose Line Is It Anyway?*, you've seen improv comedy. That type of improv, called short-form improv, employs short games with structured rules that the performers explain briefly to the audience. Another type of improv, long-form improv, is my personal favorite. In long-form improv, actors take a one-word suggestion and create a

twenty-minute play based on that suggestion. I've been an improv comedian since 2007.

Most newcomers to improv think that because it is made up on the spot, there are no rules to adhere to. However, there are a few ground rules that make improv work and flow:

- *Yes, and*: Agree with what your scene partner is saying, and then add information to it. This seems simple, but it can get challenging when you don't like what your scene partner offered.
- *Make your scene partner look like a genius*: We always want to ensure that we make our teammates look as smart and capable as possible by agreeing with their ideas.
- *Don't make anyone crazy or intoxicated*: It's hard to do a scene (or anything, really) with someone who is belligerent, nonsensical, or not working with you. If you suddenly decide that your character is going to be drunk, you put a lot of pressure on your teammates to work with and around you.
- *Avoid asking too many questions*: If you start a scene with a question, it means you haven't brought anything with

you to the table. For example, starting a scene with a question like "What are you doing?" doesn't give your scene partner any gifts of information. Instead, it forces them to do all the work. New improvisers will sometimes ask a lot of questions during a scene because they're anxious and afraid to come up with their own information.

- *Listen to your scene partner:* Listening is critical when establishing and building upon a scene. If you don't know what your scene partner is saying, you can't add to it.
- *Be present in the moment:* Focus on what is happening in your scene so that you can give all of yourself to it instead of worrying about the plot.
- *Bring a brick and not the whole castle.* Bring one or two pieces of information, not ten. If you decide what your scene is going to be about before you even go onstage, you are going to have a hard time. Your scene partner doesn't know what happened in your head, and when you come onstage with too much, they get steamrolled.

I find that the basic rules of improv often apply in real life. When you're having a conversation with a friend, the best thing you can do is listen. The second-best thing that you can do is add to what they've already said.

At some point during my career, I began to realize that my experience in improv comedy had made my work with adults living with dementia much easier. I found that I was not only quick on my feet, but I was also great at agreeing and adding on to the reality that was presented to me. The more I thought about it, the more I realized there was a

beautiful overlap between improv performance and dementia caregiving— so much so that in the summer of 2016, I paired up with a friend of mine, Chris Wright, to create an improv and dementia workshop that we developed at Steel City Improv Theater in Pittsburgh, Pennsylvania. Chris and I began writing down the overlaps between improv and dementia caregiving, and we kept coming up with more and more as we went along. The biggest overlap is a phrase we teach brand-new improvisers: "Yes, and." It is the most commonly used phrase in improv.

The ground rules for improv all make sense in dementia caregiving, as well! Let's consider these rules again, but from the perspective of using them in dementia care.

- *Yes, and:* This is related to the concept of Embracing Their Reality. All we are doing is taking what someone living with dementia says to us, agreeing, and then adding to it. A great example would be if your mother said, "I saw my parents earlier today," instead of replying, "No . . . they passed away years ago," you can say, "Yes, and— that sounds like a great afternoon." You don't literally have to say, "yes, and," but employing this strategy of agreeing and accepting information as a gift, and then adding to it, allows for a much smoother conversation.
- *Make your scene partner look like a genius:* When your "partner" is someone living with dementia, set them up for success. If you see your loved one struggling with a task, simplify the task by breaking it down into steps that they can succeed in completing.

- *Don't make anyone crazy or intoxicated:* We never want to remind a person that they are living with dementia or that something is wrong with their memory. Just as we'd treat our improv teammates with care, we want to treat the person living with dementia with care. We want to make sure they feel heard, understood, smart, and respected.
- *Avoid asking too many questions:* We never want to rely on someone's short-term memory, and typical questions usually do just that. "What did you eat for breakfast today?" is not a positive conversation-starter. Just as you would not want to hit your scene partner with a question right off the bat, we do not want to introduce a lot of questions when speaking to someone living with dementia.
- *Listen to your scene partner:* Listening is key in both improv and dementia caregiving. If you don't listen, you can't solve behavioral challenges. We always want to "hear" what the emotional issue is, and this involves intense listening, both to body language and verbal words.
- *Be present in the moment:* Instead of worrying about what will happen later, or what happened before, be present with your loved one. One of the unique things about dementia is that because it is difficult for people to recall short-term events, they are often quite present in the moment. So be present with them and celebrate the little things.
- *Bring a brick and not the whole castle:* Bring one or two pieces of information, not ten. This advice is helpful when doing activities or tasks with someone who is living with dementia.

If you give them a laundry list of tasks to do, they probably won't do any of them, because it is too confusing or overwhelming. Break tasks down into smaller steps and offer information one sentence at a time.

None of these skills come overnight, just like none of your caregiving skills likely come at first learning. All these things take practice, and I think they make the most sense when we apply them outside of dementia caregiving. I sometimes find that caregivers feel alone and stuck, as though they are experiencing all their struggles in a bubble. Care partners are far from alone, and I encourage everyone who provides care to another person to find themselves a hobby. Perhaps an improv class could be your next endeavor.

Putting It into Practice

I teach improv classes to the mild cognitive impairment (MCI) group that I work with in Pittsburgh. BRiTE is a group for adults living with MCI and early stages of dementia. We use interventions such as art therapy, music, dance, yoga, and more to improve participants' cognitive abilities. Here is a selection of the games I play when doing improv with my participants. Bear in mind that you need to adapt these exercises depending on the group size and dynamic. These are great exercises for recreational therapists or other program directors to use at their care communities or adult day care centers.

Ball Passing: Pass colored balls around the circle. Name the color of the ball when you receive it, and when you pass it. You can also draw a new number or color on the ball so that it takes extra brain energy to name what it is.

Red Ball: Use invisible balls or other items. Name each item, one at a time, and "throw" it to someone else in the group. "Red ball," you say as you receive it, and then say, "Red ball" again as you throw it. Each person repeats this as they catch and toss it.

Name Game: Each person gives themselves an alliterative, descriptive name, such as "Rambunctious Rachael." I also pair this with a hand gesture, such as mimed boxing glove hands. Say your name and do your gesture, and then pass to another person in the group by saying their name and doing their gesture. You can also do *just* names or *just* gestures.

Imagine and Describe: Think of a location, such as a dentist's office. Go around the circle and ask members questions about the new, made-up location. "What is the name of this office?" "What color are the walls?" "What's the business slogan?" Accept and acknowledge every contribution.

Pattern Game: Name any object, and ask the person next to you say something that reminds them of that object. The person next to them names another thing that reminds them of the word they just heard. And so on. "Bird," "tree," "treehouse," "fort," "battle," "skirmish."

Zip Zap Zop: Point to someone and say, "Zip!" They point to another person and say, "Zap!" Keep going with this and eventually add new words, such as Zop, Mip, Map, Mop, Lip, Lap, Lop, etc. It's important in this game to point and look at the person.

A, B, C: This game is like Zip Zap Zop but with the alphabet. To make it more difficult, add numbers, like "A," "1," "B," "2."

Clap: Try to clap at the same exact time as someone else by making eye contact and preparing for it. They turn to someone else and do the same thing.

Gestures to Numbers: Assign numbers to body gestures, such as a foot kick. Play by calling out numbers and having participants respond by acting out that number's gesture.

Birthday Gift: Pick up an invisible box and hand it to the person next to you. They will open the box and decide what's in it. Whatever they say is the right answer. Agree and tell them why you got it for them. If they say, "It's a cake!" say something like, "I ate the entire cake that you made last week, so I baked you a new one."

Yes, And: Go around the circle and use the phrase "yes, and" to create a story in the first person. You say, "I woke up late because my alarm clock was broken." The person next to you says, "Yes, and I went to the store to buy a new one." Go around the circle with each person saying, "Yes, and I . . ."

Perfect Pair: Name an item, and then the person next to you names a new item that goes with it. After that, the person next to them names an item that goes with it. You can also play this game with compound words.

Barney Sells Bread in Bulgaria: Each person chooses an alliterative word to create a silly sentence. Start by saying a person's name that starts with A. The next person says an action word that starts with A. The next person says an item that starts with A, then a location, and so forth. Allow for missteps and work them in.

Books: Each person names one word in a made-up book title. Talk about the book and ask questions about it. "When was it published?" "How much does it cost?"

Bunny, Bunny: Gesture toward yourself with two bunny-ear hands, and say, "Bunny, Bunny!" Pass it to someone else by gesturing toward them with the ears and say, "Bunny, Bunny!"

Build Sculpture: Use cut-out paper shapes to create sculptures on a table. Have everyone toss a shape or two from their hand into the circle. However it lands, it lands. Ask everyone what they see.

Ad Game: Name a common problem, like putting sheets on a bed, and have participants think up a brand-new product that will solve that problem. Ask them questions about the product and how to market it.

Picnic: Start by saying, "I'm going to a picnic and I'm bringing . . ." and then go through the alphabet, with everyone adding an item to the list while also recounting the items that came before it.

Charades: Name a group of items, such as things that you find in a kitchen, and have each participant mime an item with their hands. Let the group guess what each thing is.

CHAPTER 9

Communicating with Someone Experiencing Hallucinations and Delusions

"What are some of his symptoms?" I asked Bob's wife. "Well," she started. "He hallucinates pretty frequently." I was startled, because hallucinations hadn't been noted on any of his paperwork. "When did this start?" I asked, thinking maybe he had a urinary tract infection or another medical issue that was causing him to see or hear things that weren't there. "Oh, he's always done it, ever since his dementia began," Missy explained. "He talks about going over to his mom's house all the time, but she died ten years ago." Missy had mistaken hallucinations for delusions, a common mistake, but one that could cause someone living with dementia to receive the wrong treatment.

A *hallucination* is a sensation or perception that appears to be real but is not. A person can see, smell, hear, taste, or even feel a hallucination. For example, a person who hallucinates may see a dog in a room where there is no dog. The dog may appear and sound very real to the person who is hallucinating.

A *delusion* is a fixed, false idea, such as believing that one's mother is still alive when she passed away years earlier. You will often hear people label delusions as "confusion" or "confabulation," although delusion is the proper medical term. Delusions are incredibly common in dementia, and we expect them when we're working to embrace someone's reality.

Hallucinations

Not everyone living with dementia experiences hallucinations, although everyone living with dementia does experience delusions. However, hallucinations are common in some dementias and in other disorders, like schizophrenia. Hallucinations can also occur when people use illicit drugs or start taking new medications.

"Well aren't you just precious?" Edna asked, reaching out to touch the little boy she thought was standing next to her. But no little boy stood there. In fact, Edna wasn't standing next to anyone. Edna reached out, touched air, and smiled at us. "Could someone get him a glass of water?" she asked.

"Uh, sure," a staff member offered and went to the kitchen to fetch the "boy" something to drink. "We really need to get her checked out by a physician," the staff member whispered to me. "This is not the normal Edna I'm used to!"

———

As it turned out, Edna had a urinary tract infection (UTI). Because the staff member knew her so well, he knew when something was wrong. He recognized that Edna was not behaving normally and decided to seek medical help immediately. Thanks to his quick action, Edna's UTI was treated with antibiotics, and the infection cleared up fairly quickly. With her UTI under control, Edna stopped hallucinating.

Many people assume that a family member or friend living with dementia will hallucinate at some point. This is not true—many people living with dementia never hallucinate. Some types of dementia, though, such as dementia with Lewy bodies (DLB), are known for causing vivid hallucinations. People living with DLB are much more likely to hallucinate than people with other forms of dementia because of the way the disease affects the brain (see chapter 3).

Unless a doctor has told you that your loved one living with dementia may hallucinate, make sure that they have a full medical checkup after an episode of hallucinating. In most cases, when a person begins hallucinating, the caregiver should seek medical help quickly. Often, as with Edna's UTI, a hallucination signals an underlying medical issue. It is imperative that a caregiver doesn't write off hallucinations as a normal part of dementia.

Handling Hallucinations

Although it is important to seek medical help for someone who is hallucinating, as a caregiver, you still need to provide support while they are hallucinating. Disagreeing with them about what they see could lead to an argument. So, as always, Embracing Their Reality is critical. For example, if your loved one sees a neighbor who does not exist in the garden, be sure to agree that you also see the neighbor. Recall that what she's experiencing is real for her, even if it isn't real for you.

Hallucinations can sometimes frighten both the person living with dementia and their caregiver. In some cases, hallucinations will make it hard for people living with dementia to carry out activities of daily living. They may be afraid to sleep, eat, or walk around the house. Some people will hallucinate that bugs or animals are in their bed at night, whereas others may decide that people walk in and out of their rooms. Although challenging, caregivers must face the problem directly. Arguing with a person who is living with dementia about the hallucination or trying to convince them that the halluci-

nation isn't real will not prove effective. Hallucinations are extremely real to those experiencing them.

A client of mine had begun seeing a man outside of her living room window, which frightened her. There was, in fact, no man present, and her family tried to explain to her that he wasn't real. This didn't help, though, since she truly believed he was there. I advised the family to make a fake phone call to the police next time she saw him outside. Because they kept telling her that "no one was there," it made her feel misunderstood and probably a little crazy. "Whatever she sees, you see, too," I explained. Her husband nodded. A few days later, her hallucinations brought the scary man back to the window. "Let's go to the other room and I'll call the police," her husband reassured. This calmed her down immediately, as she felt that her husband was solving the issue.

Delusion or a Hallucination?

Families sometimes ask me, "But why does my loved one think this thing?" or "Why does my loved one hear or see this particular thing?" While there may be an answer, I remind families that it doesn't really matter *why* their loved one is experiencing a particular event, but *how* they are experiencing that event. Are they happy? Are they fearful? Just like we embrace the reality of someone who is delusional, we embrace the reality of someone who is hallucinating. I had a

woman tell me at a conference, "My mom has tinnitus—ringing in the ears—and she thinks people are constantly outside doing roadwork. If we disagree and tell her that it's just in her ears, she gets upset and calls all her neighbors to verify the origin of the sound. It's much easier if we agree that people are working on the road." No one wants to feel like they are the only ones hearing, seeing, or experiencing something.

"There he is," Terrence said, pointing at the mirror. "That's my neighbor, Ben."

Terrence's son, taken aback, watched as his father talked to the mirror.

"Hey, Ben, what's going on?" Terrence jovially asked the mirror. Terrence went on to describe how his day had been and offered to meet Ben outside their rooms for dinner. "I'll see you in a few minutes," Terrence told the mirror.

Terrence and his son walked out of the room and waited for Ben. "I'm not sure where Ben is," Terrence said, looking up and down the hallway.

Afraid of what would happen if his father waited too long, Terrence's son spoke up. "Dad, let's just head down to dinner, and I'm sure that Ben will meet us there," he said.

Terrence shrugged. "I guess so," he agreed.

———————

Thankfully, Terrence's son decided to embrace his father's reality. Terrence's brain was unable to make sense of his own reflection. He could not understand why and how he had aged so much because the man he remembered being was not that old. It made sense, then, why Terrence believed that his aged reflection was a neighbor. He created an identity and named him Ben. Terrence wasn't hallucinating. Rather, his brain was making sense out of a real situation—seeing his reflection as an old man—when what he saw didn't fit his reality. Terrence's reflection existed, but he gave it a different identity. A person living with dementia may confuse objects, light, noise, or other items in his environment for something else. For example, a large chair in the corner of a room could look like a big, hulking bear to a person living with dementia.

———————

Beth stood in the hallway and pointed, her eyes growing wide. "Look at that!" she cried out, tugging at my sleeve. "Look at those leaves falling inside."

I looked down the hall, but I didn't see any leaves. Thinking that she was hallucinating, I probed further. "Where are the leaves coming from?" I asked.

"Right there," she answered and pointed to another resident. I looked and then realized that the other resident wore a shirt covered with a pattern of falling, brightly colored leaves.

———————

Because the other resident was walking away from Beth, it looked to Beth like the leaves were moving. This was not a hallucination but a moment of confusion in Beth's mind. Dementia is a brain disease, compromising Beth's vision, perception, and spatial awareness. If Beth had seen leaves falling but the resident with the leaf-patterned shirt didn't exist, she would have been hallucinating. In this instance, however, Beth was unable to distinguish between a shirt with a design of leaves on it and real leaves.

Points to Take Away

It's important to know when people living with dementia are truly hallucinating and when they are confusing stimuli in their environment. Hallucinating could be a sign of something medical, but confusing stimuli is normal, and confusion about stimuli can be fixed easily. For example, perhaps a strained light coming through a foggy window makes it look as if another person is in the room. A dark shadow on the floor or a black rug could appear to be a hole. When a person living with dementia seems to be hallucinating, it is crucial to determine the cause.

Once you know that the person is confusing stimuli and not hallucinating, you are better equipped to deal with it. If something in the environment is the culprit, change it. In the case of the foggy window, perhaps drawing the shades would keep the room from looking as though another person was present. In the case of the black rug, removing it from the room would probably eliminate your family member or friend's fear of falling through a hole in the floor.

In summary, recall that there are major differences between hallucinations and delusions and that it's imperative we know which one a person is experiencing. While delusions are incredibly common and expected in dementia, not everyone living with dementia hallucinates. While we always want to lean into the reality of the person experiencing the hallucination, we also want to ensure that they're receiving a proper medical workup to confirm whether anything is physically wrong.

Putting It into Practice

If your loved one living with dementia appears to be hallucinating, here are some helpful steps to take and questions to ask yourself.

Ask them to describe what they are seeing, hearing, smelling, tasting, or feeling.

Keep track of where the hallucination takes place and at what time of day. Is there a connection that you can establish or something in the environment that can be changed? For example, perhaps a mirror is casting a reflection that is triggering a hallucination.

Did this hallucination begin suddenly, or has it been occurring for a long time?

_____

About how many times a day or week is your loved one experiencing hallucinations?

_____

RESOURCES

Deardorff, W. J., and G. T. Grossberg. 2019. Behavioral and Psychological Symptoms in Alzheimer's Dementia and Vascular Dementia. *Handbook of Clinical Neurology* 165: 5–32. https://pubmed.ncbi.nlm.nih.gov /31727229/.

Small, G. W. 2020. Managing the Burden of Dementia Related Delusions and Hallucinations. *Journal of Family Practice* 69: S39–S44. https://pubmed.ncbi.nlm.nih.gov /33104106/.

Williams, K. N., Y. Perkhounkova, Y.-L. Jao, A. Bossen, M. Hein, S. Chung, A. Starykowicz, and M. Turk. 2018. Person-Centered Communication for Nursing Home Residents with Dementia: Four Communication Analysis Methods. *Western Journal of Nursing Research* 40, no. 7: 1012–31. https:// pubmed.ncbi.nlm.nih.gov/28335698/.

CHAPTER 10

Helping with Timeline Confusion

For people living with dementia, time isn't linear

A recurring fear for many people who love someone living with dementia is that their loved one will eventually forget who they are. This is a frightening and disheartening thought for most anyone. How will they cope if the person they love can't remember who they are? I hear this question often and think it is important to break it down before we despair completely.

1. Hollywood has taken a lot of liberties with this narrow view of dementia for the sake of movie and TV plots. What they depict is unrealistic; a person with dementia does not always decline in the way that is often presented.
2. Your loved one does not "forget" you. Rather, it may be that they cannot place you on their timeline.
3. For people living with dementia, time isn't linear the way it is for someone without a dementia disease (Eriksen).
4. If your loved one does begin to have trouble placing you on their timeline, it won't have happened overnight. There will be a lead-up to this, and there may be moments where your loved one is more lucid than other times.

5. You are loved, you are important, you are needed, and you are not forgettable.

Tabitha cruised down the hallway with her walker. We usually called her Tab for short, and it was a cute, fitting name. Tab was a petite woman with big green eyes whose favorite outfit was a tracksuit. She was living in a moderate to advanced stage of dementia, and most of her sentences came in the form of songs. "How do ya do, how, how, how, do ya do," she sang happily, tapping her walker on the floor in time to the beat. "All right, let's go," Tab would often whisper, trying to inspire other residents to walk somewhere with her. Usually, it worked.

Tab could often be found with a group of other residents, cruising down the hallway. Those who needed some guidance had Tab. Tab was not sure where she was going, but she was going somewhere—and quickly. Tab's son Mike was often by her side. He fully embraced his mother's reality and recognized that she had cognitive impairments. Mike would come in the door and immediately inquire, jovially, about his mother's whereabouts. "Where is she off to today, I wonder?" he would laugh.

Once Mike located her, he would walk alongside Tab as she cruised the hallways, greeting new and old friends. He would sing and clap with her, and she would smile approvingly. One day, I met them both in the hallway. "Tab, do you want to come listen to music?" I asked. "We have a singer coming in to perform for us."

Tab's bright eyes lit up, and she turned to her son. "Oh yes! My husband is a great singer!" she said, pointing to her son. Tab nodded, kept walking past us, and I turned to Mike.

"I'm curious: does she often think that you are her husband?" I asked.

"No, not always," he replied, smiling. "Sometimes I'm my brother, sometimes I'm my dad, sometimes I'm me, and sometimes I'm just a friend. But always, she recognizes me. She always knows that she loves me."

_____

As Mike realized, his mother still knew him—she just could not always place him in context. She always recognized his importance to her. Although it probably sometimes pained him to realize that his mother wasn't always sure he was her son, Mike focused on the positive: Tab knew him, and she knew they had a loving bond between them. That was what was most valuable to him—they still shared a positive, happy connection. She did not wake up one day and suddenly not know him. It was not a random, sudden change. Some of Tab's days were more forgetful than others, but she always knew that she knew her son, somehow. This is what I call Timeline Confusion. *Timeline Confusion*

is the idea that someone living with dementia will know a loved one but will have trouble placing them on their timeline. For a person living with dementia, time is not as linear as it is for someone who is not living with a dementia disease.

Tab's story is quite common. What happens most often to people living with dementia is that they have trouble placing relatives and friends in context. They frequently make up, create, or *confabulate* a relationship with a relative or friend. Confabulation happens because a person living with dementia is looking to make sense of something that does not make sense to him. For example, you are visiting your father in a dementia care community, and your dad seems to know who you are, but he is having trouble identifying the relationship between you. He knows that he knows you, and he knows that you two are close. He just cannot seem to figure out *why* he knows you so well. "Who is this grown woman walking in the door?" he may think. "She sure looks like my daughter, but my daughter is a teenager. She's here, calling me Dad, but my daughter is only nineteen." When your father pictures you, he sees a young woman in her teens or twenties. Suddenly, you, as a grown woman, walk in the door. Because your father's ability to understand time and aging is impaired, he doesn't recognize you in context.

Penni is one of my favorite people. I met her during my time working with adults living with dementia. When her family decided to move her to a new community, I went to visit her. I steeled myself, realizing that she might not remember me. As soon as she met my eyes, however, a smile beamed across her face. "It's you!" Penni cried out. "How did you find me? How did you know I was here?"

I smiled and shrugged. "I just knew where to look," I said.

As we walked down the hall, Penni introduced me to her fellow residents. "This is an old friend," she said, pointing to me. "She is just wonderful." Penni looked up at me with shining eyes.

I knew that she knew me, but she could not place me.

"We were at that other place together, right?" Penni would ask occasionally. Penni knew me, she knew my face, she knew what I meant to her—she just could not place me in context. "I'm so glad you came to see me," she smiled, tears of joy in her eyes.

———

I had felt close to Penni when she lived in the community where I worked, but I anticipated that she might not recognize exactly who I was. Because she was living in a moderate stage of dementia, she was able to understand that she had known me well at some point. People in advanced stages of dementia, however, sometimes have difficulty even with this type of recognition.

Timeline Confusion among residents means that staff members at care communities should not refer to residents as Honey, Sweetie, Grandma, Baby, or other terms of endearment. "Grandma?" a resident may think. "I'm 25 years old! Who does this lady think she's talking to?"

Interestingly, people living with dementia respond best to what they were called as children. If Joan is your mother, she may not understand when you call her "Mom," but she knows her first name. Also, women who were married later in life may recognize their maiden names rather than their married ones because they were called "Mrs." only during the latter part of their lives. For example, if your mother's married name is Smith but her maiden name was Johnson, she may only answer to "Ms. Johnson." See Putting It into Practice for a list of tips to help you navigate potential Timeline Confusion.

Points to Take Away

"What if she forgets who I am?" is probably one of the most upsetting questions that a caregiver faces. We all understand that a person living with dementia believes things that aren't true (delusions) and confabulates various facts and stories. It makes sense, then, that this same individual would have difficulty understanding the passage of time and their relationship with it. Because of Timeline Confusion, a person living with dementia may have trouble placing their loved one (you, for example) on a linear timeline. But remember this important point: they have *not* forgotten who you are or that they love you.

Putting It into Practice

Tips for Coping with Timeline Confusion

- *Use their preferred name* if you aren't sure that they can identify your relationship: "Beth, it has been great visiting with you today," you may say, addressing your own mother. It can feel awkward to address your mother this way, especially if you never referred to her by her first name, but doing so can help prevent some uncomfortable conversations.

- *Listen for context clues* to find out who you are to them. For example, if your dad is talking to you about "the kids," he probably believes that you are your mother.

- *Introduce yourself or others* upon meeting. At family gatherings, it may be helpful if everyone wears a name tag. These name tags can feature superlatives or alliterations, to make them more fun. An example would be "Silly Sally." It may also be necessary to walk into your loved one's room and say, "Hi, it's just me, Rachael, coming to say hello." They could laugh off your introduction, but they may also be relieved that you announced yourself.

- *Don't quiz or force a memory* from a person living with dementia. Asking, "Do you remember my name?" or saying, "Don't you remember that I'm your granddaughter!" can be unfair and unkind to a person who has trouble recalling what they had for breakfast. While your grandmother may remember that she knows you, quizzing her about your name or your exact relationship may not go well. Understand that she may remember you as a 5-year-old, and you no longer look like the child she once babysat.

- *Focus on what they do remember* to encourage a positive interaction. One of the best things to do with someone living with dementia is to talk about things you know they remember. Focus on past events, especially things they did as children or young adults. If your loved one grew up on a farm and has fond memories of helping their father feed the chickens, then talk about chickens. If they loved going to the beach with the family, ask about the ocean.

- *Don't talk about the recent past or the present* if they aren't sure about time. It's best to avoid asking about the present unless you know that they will be able to talk about it confidently. A person living with dementia can find it confusing and painful to try and remember something that happened only a few hours—or minutes—before.

  If the present does come up, agree with their perception of reality.

- *If you aren't sure what the "truth" is, ask a staff member or someone reliable* for guidance. If you want to find out something about your family member or friend's care, it is best to ask the staff instead of relying on someone with dementia for accurate information. For example, your aunt living with dementia may or may not be able to tell you if she took a shower, ate lunch, or had her hair done. Although she may have had a soothing shower, a delicious lunch, and a great time having her perm set, she may not remember. Instead of trying to sort through her memories, talk to the staff about what she has or hasn't done that day. This will keep you from quizzing her, and you'll receive the most accurate information.

- *You're welcome to throw them a birthday party*, but if they don't remember their age, don't make it about the year: if dad doesn't realize that he's 90, don't get him a card saying, "Happy 90th!" That would be pretty confusing for him if he thinks he's turning 50.

RESOURCES

Berry, B. 2014. Minimizing Confusion and Disorientation: Cognitive Support Work in Informal Dementia Caregiving. *Journal of Aging Studies* 30: 121–30. https://www.ncbi .nlm.nih.gov/pmc/articles/PMC4443911/.

Eriksen, S., R. L. Bartlett, E. K. Grov, T. L. Ibsen, E. W. Telenius, and A. M. Rokstad. 2020. The Experience of Lived Time in People with Dementia: A Systematic Meta-Synthesis. *Dementia and Geriatric Cognitive Disorders* 49: 435–55. https://www.karger.com/Article /Fulltext/511225.

CHAPTER 11

Personal Preferences

A lifetime of likes, dislikes, and habits remain despite living with dementia

Wat someone's religious affiliation is, what hobbies they enjoy, what foods they like and dislike, who their favorite celebrities were and are—all of this information tells a story. When we gather information like this—even the seemingly trivial pieces—it provides a better picture of who this person was before dementia, and what they may need from us now that they are living with a cognitive disease. An individual's preferences are particularly important in dementia care environments because they help family and professional care partners provide person-centered care. This is why many care communities ask care partners, upon move-in, to fill out questionnaires about their family member or friend. If the community doesn't have you fill out a questionnaire, it is still a good idea to give them this information about your loved one. In Putting It into Practice, I've included a list of questions that will guide you in supplying this kind of information.

"What Did You Use to Enjoy?"

One of the most stressful parts of my job as the director of a dementia care community was working with brand-new residents whom I did not know much about. Occasionally, we'd receive a new resident admission from a local hospital late in the day. I'd go to greet them, only to realize that I knew nothing about this person other than their name and date of birth. Neither of these pieces of information told me *who* this person was as a human being, so it was difficult to provide person-centered care before I gathered other important details.

What do we do if we don't know what this person's hobbies and likes are? Individuals living with dementia sometimes experience changes in their personalities, likes, and dislikes. For the most part, however, a person's core personality stays intact, and their hobbies and likes remain. When we find out what these things are, we can apply them to who this individual is currently. I have found that asking someone living with dementia "what they like" or "what hobbies they enjoy" doesn't always tell me about them. When I've asked these questions, I usually received an answer like "Nothing" or "I don't know." Rephrasing it and asking instead, "What did you use to like to do?" elicits a more appropriate response. When you ask, "What do you like to do?" the person may think, "I don't do much of anything anymore," and answer that way. When they hear "What did you use to do?" they can reminisce and provide that answer.

Staff members will get to know the community's residents, but useful information from the family questionnaire is something they can apply firsthand to improve the resident's care sooner. For example, if the staff at a care community know before meeting your sister not to mention her ex-husband, they will not make the mistake of bringing up her marriage. If they know your brother only drinks his coffee with milk and sugar, they will not have to spend days trying to figure out why he keeps spitting out his black coffee at mealtimes. It's worth repeating that accommodating personal preferences plays a huge role in positive dementia caregiving. Providing community staff with information about your relative, partner, or friend will enhance their ability to provide good-quality care.

"Mom loves to drink coffee in the morning," Jane explained to the staff at her mother's dementia care community. "Please make sure that she gets a cup." The next morning, the staff prepared Mariah's coffee and served it to her in the dining room. Mariah was living with moderate to advanced dementia, and she was still able to use utensils and eat without assistance. She looked at the cup of hot coffee that morning and continued to eat her breakfast. "What's wrong, Mariah?" a staff member asked. "You don't like coffee?"

Mariah seemed confused by the question and continued to eat. She left the table that morning without drinking any of her coffee. For the next five days, the reaction was the same. Mariah looked at the coffee and ignored it. The staff offered her cream and sugar, hoping that would solve the problem, but she ignored this as well.

Mariah's daughter came to visit the next weekend, and a staff member approached her regarding the coffee situation. "Your mom doesn't seem to like coffee anymore," the staff member said. "We bring her a hot cup every morning, and we even offer cream and sugar. Maybe she just doesn't enjoy coffee these days."

Jane paused and thought for a moment. "Oh, mom always had a newspaper in front of her before she would touch her coffee!" she offered. "Maybe that's what she's missing."

The next day, a staff member brought in a newspaper and put it in Mariah's spot at the dining table. As she sat down, he placed a cup of hot coffee in front of her, too. A smile moved across Mariah's face as she picked up the newspaper in her left hand and began to read. Her right hand reached out and picked up the cup, bringing it to her lips.

Mariah still liked drinking coffee every morning, but she wanted it a certain way. Even though she could not communicate her preferences, once the staff met her needs, she was able to appreciate the drink. Sometimes, family members or staff assume wrongly that people living with dementia no longer want or like the things they used to enjoy. For example, if for decades your father had a habit of waking up, reading the newspaper, and then getting dressed for work, he may have difficulty getting ready for the day without the paper. It does not matter if your dad actually reads the paper—what matters is that it is an important part of his routine.

A good care community should ask a resident's family members plenty of questions about their loved one. When choosing a dementia care community, learn whether the staff gets to know residents on paper as well as in person. It should be a red flag if a community does not ask the family multiple questions about a new resident. Questions should be about a person's childhood, career, relationships, likes and dislikes, favorite foods, and potential sources of pain and trauma during their life.

The Importance of Routines

People living with dementia sometimes have trouble articulating their preferences, which may mean these preferences go unnoticed or misattributed. For example, even though your dad loves reading the paper, he may have trouble telling you that. In fact, because of his cognitive loss, he may not realize that it's missing from his routine. The newspaper cues him that it is time to get up and get dressed. The newspaper reminds him that it is time for breakfast. When daily cues are lost, so are important self-care actions. When your dad begins having trouble getting up and preparing for the day ahead, you may assume it is because his dementia has gotten worse. But the real reason is your dad is missing his newspaper—the thing that cued him to start the day. This cue, the newspaper, was a vital piece of his routine, but now that it's missing, he cannot figure out what's wrong.

When seating the residents in the dining room, I found that even a small rearrangement of the tables and chairs could throw everyone into confusion. "Where do I go?" some of my residents would ask when their seats were only a couple feet from where they used to be. Suddenly, the dining room was a new environment; no longer were things exactly where they'd been before, creating a sense for many of the residents that something was physically missing. This same effect occurs when we change an individual's routine or habits, even if we don't do it on purpose.

This is why creating and following routines is a great way to ensure that an adult living with dementia is receiving the right cues and information. When we change someone's routine, however small a change it may feel for us, we are forcing them to make an adjustment. Usually that adjustment comes with confusion or irritation, as we saw in the example of the modified dining room.

The questions a community asks about a new resident may include both personal care questions (such as about bathing and bedtime) and life history questions. Family caregivers may have difficulty answering some of these questions, especially if the primary caregiver has not lived with their parent, partner, or sibling for a long time. Before moving a person to a care community, it may be wise for caregivers to pay close attention to their loved one's routines. What time does your mother go to bed? What exactly does she like to do before she falls asleep? Taking note of these things before she needs a care community will make the move easier.

Staff members need to know what to talk to a resident about and what to avoid. This information comes from understanding their residents' personalities and life histories. History provides staff members with knowledge about a person's emotional needs. For example, knowing that a resident was a teacher for forty years tells the staff a lot about that person. It probably means that she loves kids, will try to look after other residents, and may enjoy being in charge of groups. This kind of information will help the staff plan her day and find activities to engage and interest her.

With a large group of retired teachers in our care community, we planned a trip to a local preschool to read to the children, even though all the residents had moderate to moderately advanced dementia. The minute we got to the school, it was almost as though the residents' impairments floated away.

They picked up the books the children offered and read them all, showing the pages as they went.

I chose particular residents to take turns reading to the children, careful to set them each up for success. After a couple people had taken turns, Dorothy reached for the book. "Can I read to the kids?" she asked

"Sure," I said, hesitating, afraid that she was no longer able to read. I didn't want to hand her the book if she was going to struggle with it. I didn't want her to feel embarrassed or ashamed. Even though Dorothy had been a teacher for decades, I feared that she couldn't do it any longer. Almost immediately I felt silly for worrying about it. Dorothy switched on like a lightbulb.

"Hey kids! This book is about dogs! How many of you have a dog at home?" she asked enthusiastically. Nearly all the kids raised their hands and began to get loud, trying to call out over each other. Dorothy held her hand up in the air to quiet them down. The kids stopped calling out immediately. "Wow! That is so great! Let's remember to be quiet when someone else is speaking!" she said, smiling.

Her prowess was that of an expert teacher. Dorothy read aloud to the children, pausing on every page to explain the story. The kids were engaged and excited, responding to Dorothy's cues like she had been their teacher all year. Chills ran through my body as I watched her talk to the kids that day. The children's teachers, now sitting rapt in the back of the room, had tears rolling down their cheeks. I had never witnessed anything so magical as seeing this woman transform into her old self.

Points to Take Away

We all have our own personal preferences. You can probably think of a few things that you do or enjoy that others do not. Now think about them in terms of dementia caregiving. If no one knew that you slept holding a pillow, how would you communicate this if you were living with dementia? You are having trouble sleeping, but you aren't quite sure what is different. Maybe the staff at the care community assume you have insomnia. They want to place you on a new medication, but the real solution is simple: you just sleep best with a pillow in your arms.

When I was considering all of this, I wrote my "16 Things I Would Want If I Got Dementia" list. It has gained considerable traction online, and sometimes I find people adding their own personal preferences. I wondered, "What would I want people to know about me?" and put my list together. It may be useful to make note of your own personal preferences. Write them down somewhere or type them up, and save the information in a place that others can find. If something were to happen to you, your loved ones would know best how to care for you. All your preferences would already be written down, and they would be completed by the best person possible—you.

Personal preferences do not disappear when a person is diagnosed with dementia. In fact, their preferences may become even more important. Knowing someone's daily routine and habits is vital in securing that person the best possible dementia care. The more that the staff at a dementia care community, day care, or home care agency knows about a person living with dementia, the better they are able to care for that individual.

Putting It into Practice

Here is my "16 Things" list. This is for you, the care partner: add your own items, or cross out and replace any that don't fit you.

1. If I get dementia, I want my friends and family to embrace my reality. If I think my spouse is still alive, or if I think we're visiting my parents for dinner, let me believe those things. I'll be much happier for it.
2. If I get dementia, I don't want to be treated like a child. Talk to me like the adult that I am.
3. If I get dementia, I still want to enjoy the things that I've always enjoyed. Help me find a way to exercise, read, and visit with friends.
4. If I get dementia, ask me to tell you a story from my past.
5. If I get dementia, and I become agitated, take the time to figure out what is bothering me.
6. If I get dementia, treat me the way that you would want to be treated.

7. If I get dementia, make sure that there are plenty of snacks for me in the house when I get hungry—don't wait until I ask!
8. If I get dementia, don't talk about me as if I'm not in the room.
9. If I get dementia, don't feel guilty if you cannot care for me twenty-four hours a day, seven days a week. It's not your fault, and you've done your best. Find someone who can help you, or choose a great new place for me to live.
10. If I get dementia, and I live in a dementia care community, please visit me often.
11. If I get dementia, don't act frustrated if I mix up names, events, or places. Take a deep breath. It's not my fault.
12. If I get dementia, make sure I always have my favorite music playing within earshot.
13. If I get dementia, and I like to pick up items and carry them around, help me return those items to their original places.
14. If I get dementia, don't exclude me from parties and family gatherings.
15. If I get dementia, know that I still like to receive hugs or handshakes.
16. If I get dementia, remember that I am still the person you know and love.
17. _____
18. _____
19. _____
20. _____

Here are some questions that you will want to answer about your loved one living with dementia:

- What time do they like to wake up? What is their morning routine like?
- What is a normal day like for them?
- What did they do for a living?
- What level of education did they reach?
- What was their life like growing up?
- Who were their biggest influences?
- Who was their spouse or partner? What was their relationship like? How long have they been together, and is the partner still living?
- Do they have children? How many, are they living, and what are their names?
- Are there any traumas or stressful subjects that should never be mentioned?
- What foods do they like and dislike? Beverages? Snacks?
- What is their bedtime routine like?
- At what time of day do they shower or bathe?
- What type of music do they like?
- Do they like animals? What types of pets have they had?
- What did they do for fun? What do they do now?
- What activities did they enjoy? Are there any that they dislike?
- Do they have any nicknames they prefer to be called?
- What is their sexual orientation?

RESOURCES

Alzheimer's Association. 2021. Daily Care Plan. https://www.alz.org/help-support/caregiving/daily-care/daily-care-plan.

Whitlatch, C. J. 2010. Assessing the Personal Preferences of Persons with Dementia. Chapter 21 in *Handbook of Assessment in Clinical Gerontology*, 2nd ed. New York: Elsevier. https://www.sciencedirect.com/science/article/pii/B9780123749611100211.

CHAPTER 12

Becoming a Dementia Detective

Steps for determining the root causes of dementia-related behaviors

Your parent, partner, child, or friend living with dementia will undoubtedly, at some point, exhibit unexpected behavioral symptoms. You likely have already noticed a few things. For example, your loved one living with dementia no longer wants to take a shower. Or perhaps they have begun hiding or hoarding items. No matter the behavior, there is always a root cause—and if you are patient enough, you can probably figure it out and then find a solution. *This is what it means to be a dementia detective. You need to show patience, hunt for clues, and eventually address your loved one's behavioral challenge.*

The greatest thing about becoming a dementia detective is that it takes no previous experience. You only need three things: patience, the ability to listen, and an understanding of your friend or family member's needs. Recognize, however, that becoming a dementia detective takes some practice. No one is good at it immediately, although people who have a good handle on psychology and human behavior will probably find early success. Typically, even your loved one's doctors will not be able to solve all their behavioral challenges. Some doctors may recommend taking medication, but medications can beget even more issues. As we discussed in chapter 5, although they are sometimes necessary and perhaps a good treatment for certain types of problematic behaviors, medications typically cannot solve an underlying issue caused by something environmental. As many caregivers will attest, not all doctors take the time to understand a loved one's behaviors, which means that the detective work is up to you. But don't panic! Follow along in the activity at the end of this chapter, and we can come up with some solutions together.

Understanding Their Behavioral Challenges

A little patience and a lot of trial and error can go a long way. As an example, I encountered an interesting behavioral issue at one of the communities where I worked.

"She will sit down on couches, in a chair, wherever—but I cannot get her to sit down on the toilet!" Brittany, a resident assistant, sighed. "Susannah gets really stiff and holds her pants up when you try and help her in the bathroom."

Susannah, who was incredibly pleasant, was in a moderately advanced stage of dementia. She walked throughout the community during the day, picking up objects, putting them down, and using short, sweet phrases to speak. Susannah particularly loved baby dolls and stuffed animals at the dementia care community. She would carry them in her arms, cooing gently to them.

I told Brittany to come find me when Susannah needed to use the bathroom. I was intrigued by this problem and wanted to find a solution. About an hour after we spoke, Brittany brought me to Susannah's room.

Thinking that Susannah felt uncomfortable having her pants down in front of another person, I had her hold a towel in front of her legs while I reached for her pants.

"Hmmm, yep, that's that," she said, gripping her pants so that we could not pull them down. Believing that perhaps the issue was just related to modesty, I

hoped distracting her would help. I handed Susannah her favorite baby doll and asked her to look after him for a minute. "Oh, hello," she said, smiling at the doll. This time, she let me take her pants down to her ankles while she "watched" the baby.

Brittany and I then asked her to sit down on the toilet. Susannah stiffened like a wooden board. Clearly, her pants weren't the only issue. Brittany and I tried again to get her to sit down. We walked her out of the bathroom and brought her back. We mimed sitting, hoping she would follow suit. Nothing worked.

"Do you want to sit down?" I asked Susannah.

"Hmmm, look at this," she said, misunderstanding the question and pointing to the baby. Then she said, "There's a hole."

This statement confused me at first. A hole? I wasn't sure what she was talking about. I paused, considering my options. Then, suddenly, I realized what she meant: she was afraid of the hole in the toilet.

I grabbed a bright blue towel from the bathroom wall and laid it over the toilet seat. "Hey, Susannah, sit down here," I said gently. She turned around and looked at the seat. It no longer had a hole in the middle—just a towel.

"Oh, okay," she agreed, and sat down without hesitation.

After she sat down on the new blue seat, Brittany and I gently lifted her and quickly slid the towel out from under her bottom. It was not modesty that upset her—it was the toilet itself. She was afraid of falling into the toilet bowl.

I taught this method to the rest of the care staff, who then had no more issues getting Susannah to use the bathroom.

Susannah's story provides a great example of how to put dementia detective skills to work. Although it can take some time, trial and error is the best way to solve a dementia-related behavioral issue.

Approaching Someone Living with Dementia

It's incredibly important to approach someone with dementia in the right way. Use these tips every time.

1. Approach from the front. Walk slowly toward the person you are going to greet. Do not come up behind them or tap them on the shoulder. Once you are there, meet that person at eye level. For example, if your mother is in a wheelchair, crouch beside her.
2. Speak slowly and loudly enough so that the person can hear you properly. Make eye contact and smile.
3. Use the person's preferred name and offer your hand, palm up. This will give them a chance to take your hand, instead of being touched or grabbed before they're ready.
4. Each time you approach, even if you leave for only a few minutes, repeat these same steps. You cannot be sure that a person with dementia remembers or expects you.
5. Remember that your "vibe" goes a long way. When you approach with a positive attitude, the person you're approaching will be more likely to sense this and respond positively.

Coping with Aggressive Behavior

I always hesitate to use the word "aggressive" when talking about someone living with dementia. I am sometimes asked by people who do not work in dementia care if I am ever frightened or worried about working with people in cognitive decline. It's a misconception that individuals living with dementia are "scary" or "mean." If someone does become physically or verbally aggressive, however, there are steps we can take to keep everyone safe.

If someone is becoming agitated, and it looks as though they may begin lashing out, try taking these steps to ameliorate the situation.

1. Remove other people from the area who could be injured or frightened.
2. Don't yell or threaten the person who is upset. Instead, speak slowly and calmly. Apologize that they feel badly, and suggest that you want to help.
3. Try to calmly ensure that dangerous items are out of reach, such as a chair they may want to tip over.
4. If a certain person is frustrating them, make sure that person leaves the space.
5. Give them time to regroup if possible. Ask them what they need in order to feel better.
6. If things continue to escalate, you may need to notify a person of authority. Typically, agitation doesn't last very long for someone living with dementia, and in my experience, the police are often not much help when it comes to aggressive dementia-related behaviors.
7. Do not restrain the person. Only responders trained in restraints should attempt to physically subdue the person. Once the problem is clear, it's much easier to solve.

Sundowning

Sundowning is a term that describes a common syndrome seen in people living with dementia. It describes a pattern of behavior that is exhibited in the late afternoon and evening. Although dementia-related agitation can happen any time during the day, it mostly seems to occur as the sun begins to set. Many caregivers have seen firsthand, over the course of a day, how quickly emotions can change in a person with dementia. Even the kindest, most well-tempered people can become agitated, irritable, depressed, or aggressive as the day draws to a close.

There are a few competing theories about why sundowning happens. The most likely reason is that people living with dementia—like most people—tire out as the day progresses. Throughout the day they experience stressors; deal with changes in routine, medication, and food; and interact with other people. Whereas people who are not living with dementia can announce that they are exhausted and need to be left alone, people living with dementia may have trouble expressing the same sentiment. People who are living with dementia also become overwhelmed more quickly than people who are not living with dementia. Crowded areas or loud and continuous noises can irritate adults with cognitive impairment. These limitations and sensitivities make sundowning a common syndrome, especially in care communities, where there are lots of people to interact with, a high level of entertainment and noise, and numerous visitors throughout the day.

Fear, anxiety, pain, boredom, over-stimulation, or an unmet basic human need motivates most dementia-related behaviors. I have often found that a feeling of loss precedes many behavioral challenges. This loss is often a loss of control over one's own life. It is one of the reasons you may hear a person living with dementia state incorrectly that someone is stealing from them or cheating on them—both situations bring a feeling of losing control. If you feel like you can't control anything in your life, you will probably start to panic or shut down. Some people living with dementia, unable to express their feelings any other way, will become combative or aggressive when they are hungry, tired, scared, or in pain.

Deric was becoming more and more aggravated as the day wore on. This was a normal occurrence for him. At about 5:00 o'clock each day, Deric began to pace the hallways. "Where are my mom and dad?" he would yell. Other residents would begin to get agitated, too, after hearing his cries for help.

Even though Deric was upset and looking for his parents, I guessed that there was probably another factor at play. Fortunately, it only took a couple of tries to solve the problem. "Hey, Deric, here's a snack," I said, holding out a pudding cup.

"Where are my—oh!" Deric stopped mid-yell, a smile crossing his face as he accepted the snack.

————————

The root cause of Deric's sundowning was a combination of hunger and loneliness. As soon as he was offered a snack from a friend, Deric's behavior subsided. Following an episode like this, he would typically return to his room and take a nap.

Pain and Delirium

Like most of us, people living with dementia may become more aggressive and irritable when they are tired, sick, or in pain. As mentioned in chapter 2, *delirium* is a condition that comes on suddenly and is often due to an illness unrelated to dementia. Although delirium is a treatable condition, it requires immediate medical attention because it signals that something is seriously wrong. For example, older adults who have urinary tract infections or have just come out of surgery are often diagnosed with delirium. When a person with dementia experiences delirium, he may suddenly become aggressive, confused, irritable, and even hallucinate. Recognize that delirium could be the cause of a loved one's aggression, especially if that aggression begins suddenly.

Pain tends to make people irritable. For a person living with dementia, pain can make them aggressive, in part because they might not be able to explain that they are hurting. Instead of explaining where the pain is coming from, they lash out in anger. A caregiver who fails to pay close attention may mistake this behavior for dementia-related aggression when the anger stems from physical pain.

In general, some amount of increased aggression is normal for people living with dementia. Although it's wise to prepare for a loved one becoming more combative at some point in the disease process, that change in behavior is not inevitable. Plenty of people go through the entire course of the disease without ever acting aggressively. Recall that dementia is just an umbrella term for a list of symptoms caused by many different diseases. One person's experience living with dementia will differ a lot from another's, so there is no way to predict a person's behavior as they experience cognitive loss.

My Best Tip

When we work to solve a behavioral challenge, we want to first look to see what the root cause may be. I always recommend considering that it could be a feeling of having lost control over one's life. The individual living with dementia can't do everything they used to do. While they may not be entirely aware of all their losses, they certainly recognize some of them. My best advice is to give them back some control. Ask them for help, even with simple tasks. Little things like asking, "Can you help me put these groceries away?" or "Can you help me by washing your face while I wash your legs?" will often improve their mood. Make it clear that you need them and that you know they are important. Everyone feels good when they feel needed, useful, and capable.

Putting It into Practice

I recommend making a Dementia Detective Worksheet, such as the one below. Following this example worksheet is an explanation of each step.

Step 1. Note the behavior you are concerned about.

_____

_____

_____

Step 2. Why is this behavior a problem?

_____

_____

_____

Step 3. Provide details about the behavior.
When does this behavior occur?

_____

_____

_____

Where does this behavior occur?

_____

_____

_____

What immediately precedes this behavior?

_____

_____

_____

How long does this behavior last?

_____

_____

_____

Step 4. What is the response the person receives for this behavior?

_____

_____

_____

Step 5. Describe any recent changes to the individual's environment.

_____

_____

_____

Step 6. What have you tried so far to address the behavior?
Successful:

_____

_____

_____

Unsuccessful:

_____

_____

_____

Step 7. Review the above notes to determine next steps.

_____

_____

_____

Step 1

Note the behavior that you are concerned about. Be as specific as possible. An example could be: "My client refuses to use the toilet but can usually control her bladder and bowels."

Step 2

Decide if what you are seeing is truly a problem. Is it just an inconvenience for you or the staff at the community? For example, does your loved insist on wearing pajamas all day? This could be an issue if the pajamas aren't clean, but if they are clean, it probably doesn't matter. They may just prefer to wear comfortable clothes.

Step 3

Note when and where this behavior occurs. Is it at a certain time of the day? A certain day of the week? What happens right before the behavior occurs? About how long does the behavior last?

Step 4

What happens when this behavior starts? How do others respond? For example, does everyone rush to the person's side when they get upset, or does everyone ignore them?

Step 5

What changes have happened recently to this individual or in their environment? Have they started taking a new medication? Has the senior living community been under construction or undergoing other changes?

Step 6

What have you tried so far in terms of solving the problem? Note if anything has worked, or at what general percentage each solution has worked.

Step 7

Look back over these notes. What stands out to you? If this behavior is happening only in the evening, the individual in question may be sundowning. If this behavior is only occurring when a certain person is around, could that person be causing the problem? We want to look for patterns in our notes. This may require more than one round of writing and observing, but stay vigilant! Just because something doesn't work now doesn't mean it won't work later. Most every behavioral issue has a solution, even if that solution isn't a perfect fix every time.

RESOURCES

Mace, N. L., and P. V. Rabins. 2011. *The 36-Hour Day: A Family Guide to Caring for People Who Have Alzheimer Disease, Related Dementias, and Memory Loss*, 5th ed. Baltimore: Johns Hopkins University Press.

Wojciech, R., D. Dudek, and K. Cyranka. Behavioral, Psychotic and Affective Disorders in Dementia (BPSD). In *Encyclopedia of Biomedical Gerontology*, edited by Suresh I. S. Rattan, 253–59. San Diego: Academic Press. https://www.sciencedirect.com/science/article/pii/B9780128012383114072.

Zhenzhen, W., W. Dong, D. Sun, D. Ma, Y. Zhao, H. Li, and J. Sun. 2021. Modifiable Factors Associated with Behavioural and Psychological Symptoms of Dementia among Patients Residing at Home: The Impacts of Patient, Caregiver and Environmental Variables. *Geriatric Nursing* 42, no. 2: 358–65. https://www.sciencedirect.com/science/article/pii/S019745722100046X.

CHAPTER 13

Aphasia

How do we communicate with people who can no longer use their words?

As dementia progresses, people living with it develop difficulty speaking, writing, and understanding information. The medical term for this is *aphasia,* an acquired communication disorder that impairs a person's ability to process and express language. As a care partner, you will likely find it more and more challenging to understand what a person living with dementia is trying to express. A frustration I hear from caregivers quite often is "She used to be so articulate" or "He was so well-written!" Care partners also often grieve over the loss of communication with their loved one, because they no longer feel understood. But people living with dementia continue to express themselves nonverbally. So, care partners can learn to observe body language, listen for verbalizations, understand facial cues, and watch for hand gestures to improve overall communication with the person who is living with dementia.

There is really no way to predict the entire course of a person's experience as they become aphasic. While some people will be able to communicate well throughout their life living with dementia, others will mix up words, jumble phrases, or even rely on only a few key phrases to express themselves. Some may lose the ability to speak entirely early on in the disease, when it seems as though their other faculties are still intact.

Early Stages of Language Loss

I once had a resident who would make jokes as a way to deflect from his trouble speaking and understanding. When playing a group word game—an activity that was difficult for Bruce—and his turn rolled around, Bruce would crack a joke. "Oh, well, you know what they always say, 'That's how the fish goes!'" and he would laugh jovially. I laughed, too, and smiled at him to make him feel comfortable. The joke didn't make any sense to me, but I knew that it made sense in his mind. I am not certain that he was reciting jokes entirely to "hide" his disorder, but I believe that he was somewhat aware of his issues and that humor seemed like a viable solution.

Another resident of mine was acutely aware of her language loss during her early stages of Alzheimer disease. It was heartbreaking to see tears stream down her face when she struggled to find the right word to fit into a sentence. Formerly an English teacher, Sara was clearly distraught by the changes in her ability to communicate. "Can I ask you something?" she said, pulling me aside one day. "Why can't I find the . . ." she started, tears suddenly bursting from her eyes. "The right, the right . . ." she continued.

"The right words can be really difficult to find, I know," I said, touching her arm and filling in the blanks.

"I know that I have . . . the disease . . . and I . . ." Sara continued, wiping at her eyes.

"It's okay," I assured her. "You're doing the best that you can and you're doing a great job. Alzheimer disease sometimes does this to peoples' ability to finish sentences. But you are doing a great job."

For someone with dementia, recognizing that you have uncontrollable communication problems can be distressing. Therefore, as caregivers, it is best to ignore the mistake, fill in the blanks when necessary, and continue the conversation as normally as possible. Use other clues to figure out what the person is saying. Saying something like "You aren't making any sense" will not help you or your family member or friend; it will just make them feel bad. Remember that she cannot help what is happening and is doing her best to communicate with you.

Losing a Second Language

As dementia progresses, people who have learned other languages tend to lose the ability to speak them.

Silvia turned to her table partner and friend, Emma. "Can you pass me the salt?" she asked. Emma nodded and handed it to her.

"Gracias, mi amor, quieres mas agua?" Silvia asked her friend.

"What?" Emma cried out. "What did you just say?"

"What do you mean, what did I say?" Silvia asked, startled, in her Cuban accent. "I asked if you wanted more water. What did you think I said?"

Silvia's first language was Spanish, and she was clearly beginning to transition back to her native tongue. Every so often, Silvia would answer a question, say a word, or speak a sentence entirely in Spanish. But she didn't realize that she was not speaking the same language as everyone else around her. Emma often got irritated and confused when this happened, but

Silvia would continue speaking as though nothing had happened.

Because our first language is learned early on in life, it gets stored in our long-term memory. Dementia first eats away at a person's short-term memory, although it eventually impairs a person's long-term memory, too. For people with dementia who learned a second language as a young adult or later, they will typically begin to lose the ability to speak their second language during early- to moderate-stage dementia. As the disease progresses, they will interweave the two languages and then, finally, will speak only their first language.

Language loss can be challenging for families, particularly when a person moves unknowingly from one language to another. Again, the best thing a caregiver can do in this situation is to rely on the person's other cues. Are they pointing or gesturing to something? Does the person look sad or happy? Using context clues can help caregivers deduce what someone with dementia is trying to communicate, even if the words make no sense.

Cursing

It is common for individuals living with dementia to lose their social filter as the disease progresses. This filter is what keeps each of us from saying inappropriate things. We're usually taught as children to think before speaking. But a person living with dementia may have difficulty holding back some of their immediate thoughts. The part of the brain that controls automatic language—the frontal lobe—can become damaged in some types of dementia. For example, when a woman living without dementia thinks, "I don't want any help from this obnoxious person," she may keep that thought to herself because she doesn't want to be rude. Instead, she might simply say, "No thank you." But that same woman, if she is living with dementia, has lost the filter that tells her to keep silent. She may burst out, "I don't want any help from you. You are obnoxious, and you can go straight to hell!"

When the filter is impaired, so is a person's ability to hold back racial slurs, inappropriate sexual advances, and vulgar language. The woman in the example above had learned, over time, to avoid saying hurtful things to people. But because dementia has damaged her filter, she now says exactly what she is thinking, exactly as she thinks it. This behavior can be embarrassing, especially for family caregivers. They need to remember, however, that dementia is a brain disease that impairs the way a person speaks and thinks.

Phrase Repetition

People in more advanced stages of dementia sometimes repeat one phrase as their main way to communicate. For example, caregivers may notice that their parent, partner, child, or friend has become fixated on a few words or a couple of different sayings. This is called *perseveration*. Often, these phrases do not make complete sense.

I once had a resident, Mary, who was incredibly repetitive. While she could speak in small sentences, she mostly perseverated on her son's name. "Max, Max, Max, where are you, Max?" she'd call in a sing-song voice. "Maaaax, Max. Hey, hey, Max!" even when Max was not there or even if he was right beside her, holding her hand. We came to believe that the sound of saying his name, along with the repetitive nature of it, was comforting to Mary; there was a sort of chant-like rhythm to it. One time, she was in our activity room, watching the news. A local sportscaster, Bob Pompeani, was on television. Mary finished watching the news and glided down the hallway with her walker. "Bob Pompeani, Bob Pompeani!" she called, happily. My staff and I couldn't help but chuckle at this one.

Although perseveration can get annoying at times, it's not really a behavioral problem per se. We found that by keeping Mary engaged in an activity, she was quieter and less likely to perseverate on names.

Complete Loss of Language

Some people living with dementia experience a complete loss of language. Typically, in later stages of the disease, most people lose the ability to speak at all. Some lose it much sooner, however. If this is what is happening to someone you love, do not despair. Oftentimes, the person can still understand what you are saying to them. I have told many care partners and staff members that some of my best conversations have been with residents who don't speak at all. Although this may seem strange, it's really because they are still communicating with me through body language. Even though I do all the talking, I watch their body language to see if they like what I'm saying. I have picked out music to play for someone with complete language loss and found that even when people cannot speak, they can sometimes still sing. If they cannot sing, we can enjoy the music together. There is no reason that every single moment needs to be filled with conversation. Silence can also be wonderful.

Coping with Language Loss

Even if a family member or friend cannot speak or doesn't seem to understand what you say, it is imperative that caregivers do not talk about the person as though they are not in the room. It is important for caregivers to include their parent, partner, or friend in the conversation and continue to visit even when they cannot verbally express himself. The ability to use context clues and body language is incredibly helpful when talking to a person who has aphasia. Recognize that the words a person living with dementia speaks may not match what they actually feel. It's up to you, as a care partner, to decipher what they mean. Putting It into Practice includes some steps for coping with lack of verbal language. There are additional resources at the end of the chapter that may help with communication.

Points to Take Away

We cannot fix or permanently improve a person's ability to communicate verbally, but we can change how we cope with their language loss. We can also increase the positive feelings around a visit with them when we know how best to communicate.

- *Do not assume that your loved one doesn't understand you.* Your body language and your verbal content can have a big impact. Even if they do not fully understand what you are saying, they understand that you're frustrated by the way that you are carrying your body and by your tone of voice.
- *Include them in the conversation.* If someone begins speaking about your loved one as if they aren't in the room, include them in the conversation. For example, you could say, "Yes, what do you think about that, Mom? How do you feel about the meals here today?" instead of responding directly to the person asking about your mother, as if she's not there.
- *Recognize when you need to fill in the blanks and when you can let the blanks stay blank.* Some people living with dementia get frustrated when they can't find a word, and in turn get frustrated with the person who is filling in the blank. Take a moment to see if they can find it themselves. If it seems like they want assistance, fill in the blank while continuing the conversation. For example, if they are looking to fill in the sentence "Why can't I find the right _____" you can say, "*Words can be hard to find.*"
- *Watch their body language for clues about what they want and need.* You can gather a lot of information from nonverbal communication.

- *Bring the story yourself.* If they have trouble communicating verbally, bring the story. Find something to talk about, and then dive right into it. Watch their body language to see if they like what you are talking about.

Putting It into Practice

Practice understanding your dementia care nonverbal cues and communication with a friend! Ask a friend or colleague to play the role of a person who does not speak. Set up an activity in front of you, such as a puzzle that you need to complete together. The goal here is to learn to attend to the nonverbal cues that the other person is expressing. After you spend a few minutes becoming more comfortable with silence, switch roles so that you can feel what it is like to have to communicate nonverbally.

Take notes to document the nonverbal clues your friend or colleague is expressing:

_____

_____

_____

RESOURCES

O'Connor Wells, B., and C. K. Porcaro (eds). Forthcoming. *A Caregiver's Guide to Communication Problems from Brain Injury or Disease.* Baltimore: Johns Hopkins University Press.

Volkmer, A., E. Rogalski, M. Henry, C. Taylor-Rubin, L. Ruggero, R. Khayum, J. Kindell, M. L. Gorno-Tempini, J. D. Warren, and J. D. Rohrer. 2020. Speech and Language Therapy Approaches to Managing Primary Progressive Aphasia. *Practical Neurology* 20, no. 2: 154–61. https://doi.org/10.1136/practneurol -2018-001921.

PART III
Caregiver Stress and Choosing a Care Community

Caregivers are often stuck at the "Where do I start?" phase, so in this section, I dive into the how, what, where, and why of beginning the transition from caring for someone at home to moving them to a care community. It is also useful to discuss what happens when someone still lives at home, because I find that home is where many caregivers begin to reconsider a loved one's living situation. I tackle caregiver stress and how to cope with the guilt and feelings of panic that come with caregiving. I talk about how to find a care community and when it may be time to consider one. And although it will vary depending on the location, cost of care is a worthwhile discussion.

CHAPTER 14

Caregiving Stress

The importance of taking care of yourself

I work with caregivers on an everyday basis. I talk with them on the phone, I offer caregiving advice in support groups, I meet caregivers at weddings and baby showers, I receive emails from care partners asking for help and comments on my blog posts. Everywhere, every day, care partners are fighting one battle or another. They bear an incredible amount of weight on their shoulders because they have their own lives to manage on top of caring for another person. Whether it is at home or in a dementia care community, caring for someone living with dementia can take a toll. Fortunately, there are ways to combat and cope with the stress of caregiving.

One piece of advice I always give care partners is, "Don't do this alone." People are often shocked when they hear me say this. "But if I don't care for my loved one living with dementia, who will?" they ask. I am not suggesting that you hand over care to someone else entirely,

but assistance, guidance, and support are out there, and you should make use of it. For example, calling an organization or agency for help, such as the Alzheimer's Association, is a step in the right direction. The Alzheimer's Association has a 24/7 helpline and information about their services on their website, including lists of support groups in your area. The website for the Alzheimer's Association is provided in the list of resources at the end of this chapter. There are also a multitude of free online services for caregivers that have sprung up, especially since the COVID-19 pandemic began in 2020. I host regular, free support groups online for my readers and listeners. Care partners often feel alone, as if they are the only ones experiencing the pressure and stress from caregiving. But you are not alone; there are many caregivers out there in the world who feel the same as you.

Remember: You Are Important, Too

Being a perfect caregiver does not mean devoting yourself twenty-four hours a day, seven days a week to your parent, partner, child, or friend's care. It means that you can ensure that they are safe and comfortable even if you are not physically present. This may mean bringing in a home care agency, choosing a dementia care community, using an adult day care center, or pursuing other options.

Tim had been putting his mother's care first for three years. He turned down nearly every invitation to go out: birthday parties, dinner dates with friends, exercise classes. Because he was so busy, Tim didn't really think about how unhappy he actually was. Tim accepted that this was his life, and his job was to care for his mother, Ruby, no matter how much care she needed. Because Ruby had cared for Tim when he was growing up, he believed it was his turn to do the caregiving—all of it.

Tim's marriage suffered. His health suffered. His friendships suffered. Even his children, grown and out of college, did not hear from him much, unless it was an update about grandmother's dementia. Still, Tim shouldered the weight of the caregiving, with no help from anyone else, including his own sister. Since Tim's sister lived in another city, he had become the sole caregiver. Tim was unwilling to invite a home care agency into his house or have his mother join a dementia care community.

When Tim's mother passed away, Tim was stricken with sadness, as anyone would be. He could not ignore, however, the small amount of relief he felt. Even though Tim felt terrible for admitting it, he was relieved that he could finally return to a normal life. What Tim did not expect, however, was the time that it took to piece back together a normal existence.

He had given up many nights out and phone calls with friends and family. Although it had been worth it to care for his mother, Tim wished that he had done a better job of managing his time. Perhaps if he had created a better balance between time for himself and caring for his mother, he would have been less stressed and more able to maintain relationships with other people.

The weight of caring for another person can be crushing. For Tim, the caregiving burden took all his time and energy. One thing that Tim did not consider was that his time and energy mattered, too. He probably felt the way that many caregivers do: they "come second" to the person living with dementia.

Sharing Caregiving Duties

Is a family member or friend willing to share the caregiving work with you? If the answer is yes, first check in with yourself by ensuring that you are willing and eager to accept help. If you aren't willing to accept help, and want to do it yourself, I highly recommend seeking out emotional assistance through a support group. Even though part of you may want assistance, fully accepting it can be a challenge since you are used to handling everything yourself. If you are ready to accept help, then you will also have to accept that the way your friend or family member provides help may not be exactly way that you'd like.

If you do opt to share the caregiving, get educated together on both dementia and best practices for caregiving for someone living with dementia. Sign up for a class in-person or online, attend a seminar about dementia, or find a book on the topic that you can both read—for example, this book! It's important that even if the two of you don't agree on everything, you both know how to properly communicate with the person who has dementia.

In addition, try not to make big decisions alone. If you are considering joining a care community for your loved one living with dementia, talk about this with your co-caregiver. Be as frank and open as possible. Talk about the pros and cons, and tour communities together. Part of having a co-caregiver is knowing that big decisions don't fall entirely on your shoulders. This should reduce your stress by easing your burden.

Make Time for Yourself

Taking time to exercise, eat sensibly, and engage socially are important parts of staying healthy, especially when caregiving. It is not uncommon to hear caregivers say things like, "But I don't have time to exercise" or "I don't have time to go out with my friends." Enjoying your life and making time for things you love will make you a better caregiver. Devoting all your time to caregiving and avoiding contact with the outside world will likely cause you to harbor some resentment toward your loved one with dementia. That isn't good for anyone.

I recall a time when one of my residents, Cleo, was dying. She was peaceful in her active dying stage, and we kept her as comfortable as possible. Her daughter was stricken with anxiety and anticipatory grief. At her request, we set up a cot for her by her mother's side, so that she could spend the night at the assisted living community while her mother slowly passed away. Interestingly, at the moment of Cleo's passing, her daughter wasn't in the room. It had been the only time in three days that she left the space for more than a few minutes. It made me wonder if Cleo had waited for that moment to die, as if she worried for her daughter and did not want her to see her pass. It felt to me like Cleo was saying, "Please, take care of yourself, and don't worry about me so much."

The ability to accept caregiving assistance from outside sources can provide you with emotional resources. Taking advantage of respite care, dementia care communities, or other help can give you the strength to be a great caregiver. When caregiving is not the only important piece of your life, you have more room to live. This can make caring for another person much, much easier.

Respite Care

One of the benefits of joining a dementia care community is that caregivers are able to provide their family member or friend with twenty-four-hour care without having to be at the person's side. Staff members take care of the person's physical and emotional needs, and care partners can visit as frequently as they want. Many people find that they are able to provide more positive emotional energy for their loved one living with dementia when they do not have to handle the physical caregiving.

Even if you feel it is not time to join a dementia care community, it may be time to seek extra help. For example, many dementia care communities offer *respite stays*. A respite stay allows a person to stay for a limited time in a community and receive all the benefits of being a

full-time resident. Many respite-stay residents stay full-time in communities for ten, fifteen, or even thirty days at a time. A family is expected to complete the same paperwork completed by the families of long-term care residents. You should receive the same orientation that family members of new residents receive.

Typically, families seek respite care because they need a break, are going on vacation, or are trying to decide if a dementia community is the right choice for their family member. A respite stay may give a family the information they need to decide about long-term care. It is not advisable, however, to "try out" a number of communities in a row in this fashion. People with dementia typically have trouble adjusting to new environments. Multiple moves in quick succession can be challenging for them.

Taking a Deep Breath

Care partners often ask, "How do you deal with repetitive questions from someone living with dementia? How do you handle certain behaviors when you just want to scream?" My answer is simple: take a deep breath. Take a deep breath, compose yourself, and provide the answer. Remember, your loved one with dementia doesn't mean to ask the same thing again and again.

You should also continue to pursue hobbies or calming techniques you already enjoy and utilize. In the Putting It into Practice activity, I provide a number of options. Keep in mind that what works for you may not work for someone else. If doing yoga with goats is relaxing for you, make time to do goat yoga. If running marathons is your idea of a good time, join a local running group to get you motivated for training. If reading a good book, coloring, painting, or simply taking a nap de-stresses you, make time for those things. Your health is important, and you deserve time for yourself.

Support Groups and Education

There is a good chance a support group for care partners exists in your area. Sometimes caregivers hear the words "support group" and feel guilty, thinking they don't or shouldn't need support for their own sake—they just need it for their loved one with dementia! Think of it this way: your loved one has *you*. You need someone, too.

Libraries, churches, an Internet search, or a quick call to your local chapter of the Alzheimer's Association can help you find support groups in your area. Some support groups are held in care communities but are open to anyone who wants to join. Others are held in local restaurants, libraries, or religious centers. Support groups often bring in speakers to promote education in dementia caregiving.

Sometimes, care partners want more information about caregiving but aren't sure where to look. I offer online dementia learning classes, where you can learn at your own pace. Check your newspaper for local events, such as speakers on dementia, or call your local agency on aging and ask about what is available in your area.

Additional Resources

The blog and online courses from Dementia by Day: www.dementiabyday .com

Dementia Friends USA: dementlafrlend-susa.org

Your local support group, found on AlzheimersAssociation.com

A phone call hotline, found on the Alzheimer's Association website or at 1-800-272-3900

Putting It into Practice

In this chapter we have discussed ways to ease the stress of caregiving. Working with a partner is one way to reduce the burden. Another way is to make time for yourself, so that you can recharge and stay connected to other things that are important in your life. Here we suggest some specific steps you can take to make caregiving less stressful.

Make a list of what is important for the time being, and another list of what is important for the future of your caregiving. What will happen if your loved one has a bad fall? What happens when their care needs grow? If there is a co-caregiver, planning ahead of time as a team is much easier than dealing with challenges as they arise.

1. What were some of your favorite hobbies before you began caregiving?

_____

2. Is it possible for you to still participate in those things? Why or why not?

_____

3. Is there a new hobby that you'd like to try?

_____

Here is a list of some stress-relieving techniques. Do any of these sound interesting to you?

- *Breathing.* A great tool is Breathe+, an inexpensive app for mobile smartphones.
- *Journaling.* There are some great apps for mobile devices or computers if written journals aren't your style. My favorite is called Day One.
- *Exercise.* Consider joining a gym, taking walks, running or jogging, swimming, doing aerobic workouts at home, dancing, or joining an adult sports league such as bowling or softball.
- *Support groups.* Caregiver support groups are often listed online or in local newspapers.
- *Art.* Try some adult coloring books, painting, drawing, or take an art class.
- *Music.* Consider learning to play the piano or another instrument, taking music classes, or singing.
- *Learning.* There are many online classes and apps for learning a new language, how to build websites, or how to code.
- *Other hobbies or stress relievers.* One of my favorite activities is improv comedy (see chapter 8). Other popular stress relievers include performance art such as theatre, creative writing or starting a book club, a Netflix binge, birdwatching, feeding ducks at your local park, home organizing and cleaning, visiting the local coffee shop, or shopping for new clothes.

RESOURCES

Alzheimer's Association. 2021. Caregiver Health. https://www.alz.org/help-support/caregiving/caregiver-health.

Oliveira, D., L. Sousa, and M. Orrell. 2019. Improving Health-Promoting Self-Care in Family Carers of People with Dementia: A Review of Interventions. *Clinical Interventions in Aging* 14: 515523. doi:10.2147/CIA.S190610.

Waligora, K. J., M. N. Bahouth, and H. R. Han. 2019. The Self-Care Needs and Behaviors of Dementia Informal Caregivers: A Systematic Review. *Gerontologist* 59, no. 5: e565–e583. doi:10.1093/geront/gny076.

CHAPTER 15

Guilt and Taking Things Away

I told a friend recently that a great deal of my job is helping care partners work through grief and guilt and making decisions. I find that the two emotions often go hand-in-hand. In chapter 14, we talked about the stress of caregiving and how to manage some of the grief and guilt that comes along with it. Here we discuss the guilt of deciding when it is time to make a big change in your loved one's life. The decisions you need to make are not easy: Should your loved one be allowed to drive a car? Should you take over as the health care decision maker? Often, the person you would've consulted with to make a big decision like these is the same person you are now forced to make a decision *about*. Particularly if that person is your spouse, you may feel panicked at the thought of choosing on their behalf.

When You Have to Decide

Care partners often come to me with complex, challenging situations. Perhaps they've walked into their mother's home and noticed that unpaid bills have piled up even though in the past she always paid her bills on time. Maybe they have noticed that their spouse is no longer remembering to clean expired items out of the fridge—a task that they used to complete without being asked. What should a caregiver do? Assist with these tasks? Issue constant reminders?

You probably know the old saying "Beg for forgiveness instead of asking for permission." This saying applies in dementia caregiving. If you are waiting for someone living with dementia to give you permission, you are probably going to be waiting for a long time. It is rare that someone living with dementia will give up the car keys, agree to move to assisted living, allow you to take over the bills, or let you invoke your power of attorney without a battle. It makes sense. This is a person who has been independent their whole life but now can't capably do everything they used to do. Realizing that you now need help, when previously you did not, must be an incredibly difficult feeling.

This means, then, that it is up to you, the caregiver, to take on many of the responsibilities that your mom or partner did previously. You might need to take over managing their finances, shopping for groceries, cooking and cleaning, and keeping their appointment schedule. For example, if your wife has an Alzheimer diagnosis and has started to mismanage paying the bills, you will need to take over the checkbook. She will probably insist that she can do it herself (especially if she has been paying the family bills for decades) and may get angry with you for trying to take over. This doesn't mean that you should give in and allow her to continue incorrectly paying the bills or, worse, spending money on a scam! You also may have to make uncomfortable decisions to protect their health and safety, like taking away their car keys or handling their medications. These changes will likely be made without your loved one's consent or agreement. There comes a time for every care partner to they realize they must start making decisions on behalf of their loved one. Understand that you are not "being mean" by taking over the decision-making. Although your spouse, parent, sibling, or friend may not see it that way, you are doing the best you can. Recognize that you are doing right by them; you are making choices for them that are healthy and safe when they can no longer make healthy, safe choices for themselves. Do not wait for permission to start making positive choices for them.

When we need to make a decision for someone living with dementia, I recommend using two different techniques. "Blame" the change on a doctor's orders, and tell them that the change is temporary. For example, tell your spouse that they need to move into assisted living, but it is only until the physician evaluates them again and deems them safe to live back at home. Saying "You have dementia and need to move forever" is far too much information for someone with a cognitive impairment to take in. I'll cover this in more detail later in the chapter and in the Putting It into Practice activity at the end of the chapter.

When It's Time to Stop Driving

Elaine shook her head. "He's not going to like that—at all," she said. We were in a care partner support group discussing the painstaking task of taking away someone's ability to drive. "He loves his independence," Elaine said of her husband. "He's going to have a complete meltdown if I try to take those car keys away from him. He's going to blame it on me, and it's going to be terrible," she uttered, putting her forehead in her hands. The rest of the group nodded in empathy. "I have the same problem with my wife," one of the men spoke up. "Is it really that bad if I let her keep driving? She's been okay so far, and she only goes to the store and back. She never gets lost!"

I often tell caregivers, just because your loved one has "been safe so far," it does not mean they will continue to be safe. It is naive to assume that just because they "don't get lost" they are safe to drive. Driving a vehicle involves more than the ability to get from point A to point B. You need good reaction time, sound judgment, an ability to recall what street signs mean, and much more. Even if someone knows how to get to the store on a map, they may not be able to do it *safely*. Think about it this way: If you wouldn't let your loved one living with dementia drive with a child in the car, should you be letting them drive at all? They could get in an accident and hurt themselves, another driver, a cyclist, or someone walking down the road. And in some states, if you are the primary caregiver, you could be opening yourself up to legal liability if they are in an accident. Please consult an attorney to find out about the laws in your state.

When is it time to take away the car keys? The answer is as early as possible. When a physician makes a dementia diagnosis, it's also a good time to start the conversation about no longer driving. If the person begins to get lost, drives dangerously, ignores road signs, experiences a loss of reaction time, has faulty judgment, or seems confused about how to start or stop a vehicle, it is absolutely time for that person to stop driving. Of course, preventing a person from driving is much more challenging than noticing that they shouldn't be driving in the first place.

Although some people living with dementia may agree to stop driving, expect them to put up a fight. An adult child or a spouse saying, "You cannot drive safely any longer" likely will not convince them. Most people do not want to be told to stop driving, especially when they have been driving for decades. For many caregivers, getting another party involved is the best way to stop someone with dementia from operating a vehicle. See Putting It into Practice at the end of the chapter for a how-to guide. Next, let's look at how Embracing Their Reality can defuse a difficult question, such as "Where are my car keys?"

It was getting dark outside, and Lisa felt like it was time to leave. She believed she was staying in a hotel, even though she was really just sitting in her dementia care community's common area. Lisa looked at her watch. "Eight o' clock?" she asked, mystified. "Where did the time go? It's getting late, and we should be going."

Lisa reached over to the side table to look for her car keys. "Where are my keys now?" she asked.

"Oh, Lisa," I offered. "I forgot to tell you that I took your car to the shop today. Something was wrong with the motor, and I wanted to make sure that we got it fixed for you." This wasn't true in our reality, of course, because she hadn't driven in years.

"Oh, really?" Lisa asked. "Well, thank you for getting that fixed. I guess we can just stay here another night until it's ready to go."

Different techniques will work for different people. The approach that I used with Lisa will not work for everyone. If your mother asks about her car keys, perhaps you can suggest they got lost somewhere in the house. Maybe the car has a flat tire. Perhaps someone is borrowing the vehicle for the afternoon. No matter what, recall that embracing the reality of the person living with dementia is key to a productive outcome, and re-orientation is never the answer. "Mom, you can't drive anymore, remember?" is a statement that starts a fight—not ends one.

The Guilt of Moving Someone

Deciding to transition someone into a care community is one of the most difficult decisions you will make as a care partner. There are probably a lot of people telling you what they think you should do, or what they think your loved one living with dementia "would have wanted." At some point, it is no longer up to the person living with dementia—or that pesky neighbor with a lot of opinions. Asking mom if she "wants to move to assisted living" will most likely result in a "no way." It is common for care partners to tell me that they've been wanting to join a dementia care community, but their loved one keeps saying they don't want to move. Again, dementia is a beg-for-forgiveness group of diseases. If you wait for permission, you will never stop waiting.

Step one in moving someone to a care community is getting past your *own* guilt and fear regarding the move.

When you continue to shoulder the burden of guilt, you make caregiving harder than it already is. You did not give your loved one dementia. You did not want to move them to a care community before it was time. You are not doing this because you are a "bad person" or because you are "lazy" and don't feel like caring for them at home. You are making the decision to move them because it is the safest and healthiest decision for both of you. In chapter 16, we review the reasons that you may be considering a care community setting for your loved one, or perhaps the reasons why you have already moved them. I often tell care partners, "Do not lean on your guilt as a reason why you shouldn't or can't move someone into a care community. If you are making a safe, healthy decision for both you and your loved one, you are doing the best that you can."

Putting It into Practice

Here are some tips when it comes to making decisions for your loved one living with dementia:

Recognize when they can no longer make safe decisions. Ask yourself if you'd let your loved one take over some of your responsibilities. If the answer is "no way," then we can recognize that the individual may not be able to do their own tasks, either.

Invoke the "grandchild test" when it comes to driving. If you wouldn't let them drive with their grandchildren in the car, don't let them drive a car at all.

Don't wait until something bad happens to make a change. For example, do not wait until the electricity gets shut off to assume responsibility for paying the bills. Don't wait for your loved one to get in a car accident to decide it's time to take the keys.

Don't rely on warnings or notes. Don't put notes around the home, such as reminders on doors that instruct them not to leave the house. Don't scold or warn them about doing unsafe things, like using the basement stairs. Instead, we need to find reliable ways to keep them safe that don't depend on their judgement.

Trust your gut feeling! Listen to your immediate, gut feeling—there is always weight to it.

Journaling can be a helpful and stress-relieving exercise. When we write our thoughts down, it helps us process and think through big decisions. Here, I want you to work on journaling through feelings of guilt.

1. What is something you feel particularly guilty about regarding your loved one living with dementia?

_____

2. Is this something that you have power over? For example, if your loved one is acting in a manner that you don't like, do you have the power to change it? Perhaps not.

_____

3. What can you do about this guilt? For example, could you talk to a friend in a similar situation? Maybe join a support group? Could you try mental health counseling?

_____

4. What *will* you do about this guilt? Recognize that holding on to guilt is not healthy or productive. An example would be to join a support group.

---

5. What decision needs to be made? Do you need to decide if you will move them to a care community, for example?

---

6. Can someone else help you to make a tough decision, so that it is not entirely on up to you? Who is that person?

---

7. Ask for help. Write down the name of a person or organization to whom you can turn for assistance.

---

8. Remind yourself that you are doing the best that you can. Your choices are not selfish, and you are making healthy choices to assist your loved one living with a cognitive impairment.

If you need to take the car keys from a person living with dementia, taking these steps can help.

Involve a physician. One popular technique to prevent a person from driving is to involve a doctor. Tell the doctor ahead of time that your family member should probably not be driving any longer, and the doctor can help make the official call. Hearing the bad news from a doctor may be a lot easier than hearing it from you, the caregiver. This will also prevent your loved one from taking out their anger on you.

Have a physician refer them to the Department of Motor Vehicles. A physician can refer a patient to the DMV. Your loved one can retake the driver's test and—hopefully—have their licensed revoked.

Call your local fire or police department. Many local agencies have programs that help stop people living with dementia from driving. An officer can pull your family member or friend over and require a driving test. Since it was law enforcement that made the call, if they are angry, the blame won't fall on you. The most important thing is that your family member or friend is safe and no longer behind the wheel of a vehicle.

Blame it on the car. Suggest that the car has stopped working, and that you need to take it to the shop. This mostly works with people who have poor short-term memory. You can give the car away or sell it. When they ask, "Where is the car?" remind them that it is "at the shop."

Find out where they need to go, and offer an alternative. Offer to drive them, call a car service (Uber, Lyft, or taxi, all acceptable options for people with mild cognitive impairment), or arrange a carpool with friends. If they always go to a coffee shop in the morning with friends, can one of the friends pick them up? It won't seem forced or inconvenient to stop driving when they have a free ride.

CHAPTER 16

How to Handle Family Dynamics When Choosing a Care Community

Managing expectations and unwanted input from relatives

I talked to Uncle Rico on the phone last week, and he seemed just fine," Vanessa argued. Vanessa's cousin Maribel had recently moved her father, Vanessa's Uncle Rico, into a dementia care community, but Vanessa didn't think it was a good decision. "We talked for a half hour and his memory was great! He doesn't belong in one of those places," she stated.

Although Vanessa only wanted the best for her beloved uncle, she was missing a few crucial pieces of information. For starters, Maribel had been her father's primary caregiver for the past two years. The stress of his progressing dementia was tearing Maribel apart. She'd hired a caregiver to come to the house four times a week, but the caregiver had quit abruptly last month.

Maribel had her own children to contend with, let alone her father's declining health. Also, while Vanessa was focused predominately on her uncle's memory, there were other issues at play: his ability to toilet and bathe independently, his constant need for medication reminders and mental stimulation, his ability to make safe decisions regarding his own care.

After touring a couple of communities and talking to a placement agency for assistance, Maribel chose a place she thought was best for her dad. It crushed her that Vanessa doubted her choices. "What if I made a mistake?" Maribel asked herself in the car outside her dad's dementia care community. "Maybe Vanessa is right. Maybe dad doesn't belong here yet," she sighed to herself.

Having Confidence in Making the Hard Choices

Remember, we cannot sit and wait for a person living with a cognitive impairment to make safe decisions for themselves. I have occasionally met family members of those living with dementia who say, "My spouse doesn't want to move to dementia care" or "My father doesn't want a home care agency to come in and help him just yet." A person living with dementia who needs help is most likely not going to recognize that they need assistance. Unfortunately, it falls on the care partner to decide what to do with regard to their loved one's care.

Making tough decisions is a difficult challenge for many caregivers to overcome. In fact, I meet plenty of people who never overcome it. Instead, they choose to do nothing regarding their loved one's care. The person living with dementia ends up living alone, often without the assistance they require, because the individual's care partners felt uncomfortable taking health care choices away from them. Situations like this never end well for anyone. Choosing to not do something because you fear offending or upsetting the person living with dementia is actually setting the individual up for failure. Just because they won't like the choice that you are making does not make it a bad choice. If you are looking out for their safety and well-being, you are making the best choice possible.

Above all else, remain confident in your choices. In the above story, we saw how Maribel's cousin questioned her choices regarding Rico's care. Although Maribel may have previously felt positive about her decision to move her father, Vanessa's insistence that it was the wrong decision made Maribel question what she had done. In this story, like many other stories I have watched play out in front of me, Vanessa was not present for her uncle's progressing dementia. Although Rico may have "seemed fine" to Vanessa during a thirty-minute phone call, Maribel knew better. Maribel saw her father's declining health up close, and she knew that he needed more care than she could provide. Though Maribel's confidence was shaken, she eventually realized that she'd done the right thing by moving her father. He was well cared for and safe in his care community. This was more than she could have provided, around the clock, in her own home.

Denial, Guilt, and Anxiety

If you are reading this book, you may be the primary caregiver to someone living with dementia. Perhaps you are lucky, and your siblings, friends, or other members of your family are integral to your loved one's dementia care, providing help and assistance when you ask for it. More likely, however, you are one of many care partners who feel alone and isolated in your caregiving journey. If this strikes a chord, recognize that you are not alone. When I host support groups or family training workshops, I always stop and ask my audience to look around the room. "Everyone in this room is going through the same thing," I say. "Maybe their stories are slightly different from yours, but they feel a lot of the same pressures and anxieties that you do. You are never alone in your caregiving journey, even if other members of your family or close friends do not provide you with much support."

It can be a real challenge to remain confident and steadfast in your caregiving choices, particularly if someone close to you doesn't think you're making the right decisions. They may make comments about how you're "doing the wrong thing" or question what you have done. It is easiest to make choices for someone else's care when you obtain the paperwork for durable power of attorney. In the story earlier in this chapter, Maribel was her father's medical power of attorney, so she had the final say about what happened with her dad's care. Your own story may be more complicated. It may be that you share power of attorney with a relative or friend. Perhaps your entire family wants to be involved when it comes to making a big decision regarding the individual living with dementia, but no one can seem to agree on what that decision should be.

I once met a family who couldn't decide about their mother's long-term care plans. The family was made up of five adult children, most of whom did not speak to one another. Fortunately, the family had decided that since they could not agree—or stand to be in one room together—they should hire a legal guardian to make decisions on their mother's behalf. Each of the five children wanted what was best for their mother, but they realized that they would never agree on what that actually was. Something like this may be an option for you and your family if there is constant tension and arguing over the best course of action. Hiring a proxy may be best if otherwise no positive moves or choices would be made.

Hopefully, this is not the case for you. I hope you have no one in your life who disagrees with your health care choices for the person living with dementia. If you do, though, recognize that the person you're arguing with may have the same feelings about the situation that you do. Even if what they are doing or saying is completely wrong, the way that they are feeling is probably similar to how you feel: anxious, fearful, confused, and perhaps a little guilty. If the individual in question is a long-distance caregiver, they may feel guilty that they aren't with the person who is living with dementia all the time. This guilt takes the form of anxiety, which means that they pressure you, the nearby care partner, in a way they may not otherwise. This person's feelings are legitimate, even though they may be expressing them in an unhelpful way.

Take, for example, the case of Allie and her mother, Irene. Marc, Allie's father and Irene's husband, was living with Alzheimer disease. Allie was an amazing care partner for her father because she really understood positive dementia care communication. She had been to a couple of my workshops and read every book and article on dementia that she could find, all of which provided her with the skills she needed to embrace her father's reality. When Marc asked where his dad was, Allie embraced his reality, and, knowing that he believed he was at work, Allie would reply, "I think you told me that he's at work."

Although Irene meant well, and loved her husband dearly, she had a much more difficult time with the concept of embracing his reality. She felt anxious and concerned for her husband's care and didn't like to "lie" to him about where his father was. "Your father died years ago, Marc," she'd sigh. "Remember? We visited his gravestone just last week." Allie and Irene were beginning to bicker about what to say to Marc and how to handle his increasing confusion. "My mom wants the best for my dad," Allie told me. "Unfortunately, she's just having a really hard time embracing his reality. What can I do to help her?"

Isolation

It may come to a point where you feel as though you have tried every trick in the book to get this individual to understand how to provide better dementia-positive care. Instead of listening, reading, or understanding, however, they argue with you, or worse, with the person living with dementia. You hear them from the living room, arguing on speakerphone with your father. "Don't you remember? You have six grandkids! How could you forget that?" they shout into the phone.

You have tried your best to get them to understand dementia caregiving, but it does not seem to be working. In a scenario like this one, although it seems harsh, it may be necessary to isolate them a little bit from the person living with dementia. For example, if your cousin constantly starts fights with your father at holiday gatherings, perhaps you can find a way to keep them from talking one-on-one. You don't need to be threatening, such as saying, "If you can't improve your communication with my dad, I won't let you speak to him," but it may be useful to keep their communication to a minimum. We have to look out for the individual living with dementia and their well-being, even if the person they are talking to is a beloved relative.

Recognize when you yourself have had enough. It's not fair to you, the main care partner, to endure constant battles with a person who thinks you're making the wrong choices. It may make sense for you to take time away from the individual who is fighting with you. Dementia caregiving is hard enough without also having someone fight us on every decision we make.

Education

As I explained to Allie, a little education goes a long way. Most people don't know what they don't know, which means that they may not realize that the way they're approaching dementia care is not helpful. They've learned that lying is a bad thing, and telling the truth is always appropriate. Telling a loved one living with dementia their parents are dead, then, seems like the right thing to do. It may not have occurred to this individual that there are better options.

Putting It into Practice

Here is what I recommend when it comes to talking with family members who are stressed and confused with regards to dementia care.

Lead by example. We have a saying in improv comedy, "Show, don't tell," which means that instead of talking about what we are doing or going to do, we act it out. This skill applies in dementia care as well. Take, for instance, Allie's situation. She might say, "Mom, do you feel like you get into arguments with dad? I have been using a new technique, and I think it works really well," and then demonstrate it the next time he asks where his parents are. Irene may see that Allie's approach works a lot better than her own. Even the most stubborn individuals can learn by this show-and-tell methodology. They hear about a technique and then see it in action, working well.

Attend a workshop or seminar together. See if there's a dementia care workshop or event happening in your area that the two of you can attend. I have had families say to me, "My family member doesn't believe me when I talk about dementia, but they will definitely listen to an expert!"

Join a support group together. A support group is a great way for everyone to feel heard, understood, and, most of all, not alone. The Alzheimer's Association, among other groups, has resources about support in your area.

Try couples or family counseling. Particularly if your spouse or partner doesn't understand dementia care, couples counseling may be a smart choice. It's helpful to have a sort of "referee" or a neutral party to bounce ideas off of. Family or couples counseling also allows everyone to talk about their feelings on the subject, which can help families move forward together.

Give them books and articles when you can. If you believe that the other person is open to reading up on the subject, sending books or articles is a great idea. If they aren't much of a reader, try sharing podcasts, audio books, or even documentaries about dementia.

Which steps do you think are best for your family?

RESOURCES

Alzheimer's Association. 2021. Support Groups. https://www.alz.org/help-support /community/support-groups.

Kenny, A. 2018. *Making Tough Decisions about End-of-Life Care in Dementia.* Baltimore: Johns Hopkins University Press.

Lindeza, P., M. Rodrigues, J. Costa, M. Guerreiro, and M. M. Rosa. 2020. Impact of Dementia on Informal Care: A Systematic Review of Family Caregivers' Perceptions. *BMJ Supportive and Palliative Care* Oct 14: doi:10.1136/bmjspcare-2020-002242.

CHAPTER 17

Myths about Care Communities

"No one can have mirrors, scissors, or butter knives"

I walked into the skilled nursing facility's dining room just as their residents had started to eat lunch. I watched as one of their residents struggled to butter his bread with a spoon. My eyes scanned the room, noticing similar issues everywhere: people trying to cut with forks, people attempting to apply jams and jellies with spoons. I sighed. "Why do none of these people have knives?" I asked, already aware of the answer. The nurse taking me around for a tour looked surprised. "Well, they all have dementia, so they can't have butter knives," she said. "Why?" I asked her. She paused and thought about it. "I guess . . . I don't know," she answered honestly. "That was always just what the adminis-trators told us to do: take the butter knives away!"

An annoying, albeit common, practice of care communities is to take away residents' butter knives, scissors, mirrors, flowers—and the list goes on and on. Someone somewhere heard that people living with dementia would hurt themselves or others with certain objects, and therefore those objects must be hidden away. Myths like this one have been propagated throughout health care for years. Unfortunately, many of these myths are stigmatizing and damaging to the way that we treat people living with dementia. They cause us to take things from them for no good reason. They cause us to treat people living with dementia in demeaning, infantile ways.

Possible Myths

Butter Knives

People do not get dementia and suddenly turn into devious criminals, hoping to injure their tablemates with butter knives. As I often tell care community staff members, "A fork is just as danger-ous as a butter knife." Not only is a butter knife not truly dangerous, it is also unfair to take knives away from resi-dents living with dementia. Imagine that you've been using a knife to butter your bread since you were six years old. You recently moved to a new home where you eat lunch with a bunch of new people. At meals, you are supplied with a fork and a spoon. You're now in a new environment with new people and you've been handicapped with a lack of proper utensils.

I would not shy away from other types of knives, either. Unless the individual can no longer safely use a knife, or in the rare circumstance seems as though they may hurt themselves or someone else, knives are appropriate for people with dementia to use. Taking something from an entire group because one person cannot use the item is unreasonable. These are adults we are working with, not preschool children.

Scissors

Scissors are similar to knives. This individual is not suddenly a criminal; why did we take their scissors away? I often see activity directors and recreational therapists opt for child-safe scissors from craft stores. These scissors are tiny, blunt, and usually colorful—in other words, they look like they were made for children. People living with dementia are not children: they are adults who have lost some of the gains they made as adults.

Mirrors

It is a common myth that all people living with dementia will be upset if they catch a glimpse of their own reflection in a mirror. The concern here is that someone will believe they are much younger than they actually are, see themselves as an older person, and become scared or confused. Although I always tell staff members to embrace the reality of people living with dementia, this mirror myth takes it a little too far.

In all my time working in dementia care environments, I have only heard of one person being upset by their reflection in a mirror.

This is another scenario where, if an individual has an issue with the object, remove the object from their space instead of taking it away from everyone. Have you ever been in a public restroom that lacks a mirror? It's jarring! You're washing your hands and look up to see—nothing. I believe it would be more disrupting to not see a mirror than to see a reflection that doesn't quite make sense. In my experience, people who see their reflection often accept it, disregard it entirely, or even believe that an older friend or family member is standing with them.

Floral Arrangements

"They are going to eat the flowers!" I've heard on more than one occasion. Again, if one person has a habit of putting flowers in their mouth, remove the flowers from their room or dining table. Even in very late stages of dementia, most people do not look at flowers and consider eating them. We don't want to take beautiful arrangements from everyone's tables because we have a fear that one resident will ingest them. It would take a great deal of table-friendly flowers to make an adult human sick, anyway.

Glass

Can a senior living community use glass vases for flowers? Can residents keep glass figurines in their rooms? The answer is: it depends. It depends on the location and the licensure of the senior living community. For example, most skilled nursing facilities do not allow glass. This is because of the fragile nature of glass and how dangerous it is if it shatters.

Interactive Wall Art

I have been to many communities where they feel proud and excited by their wall art. "Residents can turn this wheel, unlock this padlock, turn this, touch this, and more," the man giving me the tour said. In my experience, people living with dementia almost completely ignore interactive wall art. I encourage communities to include art on the walls that makes sense and looks great, but it's more for the overall aesthetic and feel of the community than for use by residents.

Locked Units

"Why do residents need to be locked into these places?" the speaker asked the audience. "They aren't criminals! They deserve to be able to come and go as they please," he continued. It was clear to me that this man didn't have a lot of experience in health care, at least not dementia-specific care. If he had, he would have known that there is a reason we keep dementia-specific communities secure: safety. This is not to say that all such communities are secured—they aren't—but having worked in an unsecured community, I can tell you that it was a trying experience. I spent a great deal of my day rushing down the hallway, running outside, going on the elevator, all to retrieve my residents who had left the dementia-specific space. It was a huge time waster and morale killer for residents: they left, we followed them, we brought them back.

As it turned out, the man presenting *was* new to dementia-specific care. It was his first year, and he'd never actually worked in a care community. He was selling an idea, but the idea wasn't based on any actual research or experience on his part. In the unsecured community where I worked, I devised a unique way to keep my residents from exiting. I got a local vocational high school's graphic design program to design for us a decal of a bookshelf. This large sticker covered the door, and while it could still open and shut, the door looked as though it was no longer an exit; it just looked like a bookshelf. Residents immediately perceived it as such and stopped using it.

Mixed Units: Residents of Different Abilities

In this same forum, the presenter suggested that residents should all be together, regardless of their cognitive abilities. I immediately thought back to one of my first residents, Carrie. Carrie was sweet and friendly, but she was being bullied by some of her fellow residents in assisted living. She had begun having issues finding a dining table, locating her room, participating in activities, and chatting with friends. Because of her dementia, some residents that used to treat her with kindness began exiling her from their tables and programs. They were probably doing this out of fear for their own cognitive abilities, but what they were doing was mean and hurtful for Carrie.

Carrie's story is not the only one about people of diminished abilities being bullied by fellow residents. Although it sounds great to "keep everyone together," it doesn't make sense when actually implemented.

Key-Entry Doors

I have often heard families complain that their loved one "needs a key" so that they can keep their room locked during the day. Although this is sometimes possible, depending on the community, it is not easy. Many people living with dementia cannot manage keys, so they often go missing or unused.

The concern that families have usually comes from other residents entering their loved one's room and taking things. As I've told many families, that's dementia care. It is not possible to completely prevent items from going missing or being taken by other residents. For anyone who stays at the care community, that place is their home. In that way, the entire space feels as though it belongs to them, so in and out of rooms they go. Locking each door causes more difficulties than it solves.

Locking Items Away

It is true that dementia-specific communities need to lock up items that could be hazardous. Although it depends on the community, these items usually include shampoos, soaps, cleaning products, toothpastes—anything that could be potentially harmful in large doses.

Families sometimes get frustrated by this policy, but it's for the safety of the residents who live in the community. There is a difference between a bottle full of shampoo and a butter knife. Sure, you could go after a person with a butter knife out of malice, but the likelihood of that happening is very small. What is more likely is that a person living with dementia will mistake a shampoo bottle for a bottled beverage. I wish I could say I'd never heard of anything terrible like this happening, but I have. It's quite possible that a mistake in judgment could lead to serious consequences.

Points to Take Away

This chapter has covered a few of the myths and truths you may hear about dementia care. Other myths about dementia are propagated by Hollywood. Think about it: when you see television shows or movies with a character who has dementia, what are they doing? They are likely portrayed sitting in a chair, staring out a window in a run-down nursing home. Myths about what is true regarding dementia care tend to stick around for years. I've had people ignorantly ask me if places I consult with are like *One Flew Over the Cuckoo's Nest*.

If you encounter something that surprises you, stop and think about it. Ask why the community is doing this or doing that. If the answer is, "Well, we've always done it this way!" maybe it's time for a change. As we continue to get better at dementia caregiving, what we expect from care communities will evolve.

Putting It into Practice

Make a list of myths that you may have heard about memory care communities that aren't covered in this chapter. Do you have questions about what you wrote down? Check in with a knowledgeable team member at your care community, or reach out to my team directly at hello@dementiabyday.com.

_____

_____

_____

RESOURCES

Fazio, S., S. Zimmerman, P. J. Doyle, et al. 2020. What Is Really Needed to Provide Effective, Person-Centered Care for Behavioral Expressions of Dementia? Guidance from the Alzheimer's Association Dementia Care Provider Roundtable. *Journal of the American Medical Directors* 21, no. 11: 1582–86. https:// www.sciencedirect.com/science/article /pii/S1525861020304199.

CHAPTER 18

At-Home Safety

Safety precautions to put in place and things not to do

Safety at Home

Before the onset of their disease, many people living with dementia lived at home, either alone or with a partner. Most of these individuals did not stop to create a "what-if" plan for themselves if they were diagnosed with dementia. They most likely assumed they'd finish out their life living in their own home. After receiving a diagnosis of dementia, however, everyday tasks become more challenging. Your loved one may not be bathing as often as necessary, or perhaps they aren't keeping the fridge free of old food. Commonly, a family member—usually a spouse or adult child—takes on the responsibility for most of the chores around the home. Maybe the person living with dementia moves in with a relative, or maybe a relative moves in with them.

I had a man ask me recently, "How do I know when I need to move my mom into a dementia care community?" He described a situation where she was at home, safely receiving twenty-four-hour care. I indicated to him that he need not worry about moving his mom if things were working out. If she was safe in her house, he did not need to consider moving her to a care community. It's not a bad idea to have a plan in place if your loved one's health condition takes a turn for the worse, I reminded him, but if all was well at home and she had full-time care, he needn't be worried about relocating her. In this man's case, twenty-four-hour home care was working well. She lived in a ranch house, so there were no stairs to worry about. She had plenty of hand railings to grab onto, and the floor was free of clutter.

In many cases, however, home is just a starting point for care partners looking to provide the best possible care for someone living with dementia. After a while, though, home begins to present other challenges: perhaps a physical ailment limits mobility up and down stairs, a hoarding problem causes mass amounts of clutter, or the home care agencies the family has tried haven't provided adequate care.

Still, joining a care community right away isn't always a possibility. There could be a waiting list at the nearby dementia care community, or the financial cost may be too great to start care until another few months go by. Whatever the case, there are important aspects to consider while keeping someone living with dementia at home safely.

What Doesn't Work

"We have a system for him," Helena nodded, leading me into her kitchen. "See, here's his calendar. Every time he takes his medication, we mark that down. And then when he showers, that's here in blue. So now he can look at his calendar and remember when he did things." While this was a valiant effort, one I had seen countless times before, it did not work. Helena's father didn't look at his calendar, or if he did look at it, he wasn't sure what it meant. Helena and her siblings were relying on reminders and reorientation to try and help their father get through his day without incident. These reminders did not solve the inherent problem, which was that his disease had caused his judgment and comprehension to wane.

Keeping your own notes for personal record-keeping or to share with another caregiver can be helpful when used as an internal system. For example, many care partners coordinate in-home care with hired caregivers through notebooks and charts. But we never want to rely on notes left around the house to remind someone living with dementia to stay safe. Notes like, "Dad, don't go outside, you're retired and don't have to work today!" or "You're 97, this is your home, you don't need to worry," seem loving and kind. They come from a good place. A care partner wants to help a confused individual reorient themselves and not get into a dangerous situation, like trying to walk down the road alone. It is imperative to understand, however, that notes do not work. For a note to work, it would mean that the individual living with dementia would have to notice the memo, read it, comprehend its meaning, do as instructed, and then remember later what that note said. It is highly unlikely that a person with a cognitive disability is going to be able to do all those things. Relying on notes to keep someone safe in their house is *not* a safe practice.

Caregivers should also not rely on false promises to keep someone safe at home. "I told my wife she isn't allowed to use the microwave when I'm not home," a care partner once told me proudly. "So I think it's fine." Making your loved one promise to do or not do something is not a safe bet. Although there could be a chance that they disobey you just for the sake of making their own choice, there is a greater likelihood that your loved one will not remember the promise they made in the first place.

We also never want to rely on the status quo to keep a person safe. What does this mean? It means that just because your loved one has been safe at home thus far, there is no guarantee that they will continue to be safe. "Well, they haven't left the house yet" or "So far they haven't left the stove on" is far from a confident guarantee that these things won't happen. While we want to hope for the best, we also want to plan for the worst. Relying on the status quo means that we are hoping for the best without any further thought on the matter.

What Works

What *can* we do to help someone living with dementia stay safe at home? Most importantly, people living with dementia should never live alone. There is no substitute for human caregiving at this current moment in time. We will address technological advances in a later chapter, but all the apps and artificial intelligence and cameras in the world cannot currently act as a substitute for having a caregiver in the home. This caregiver may be you, it may be a friend or relative, it may be someone from a care agency you have hired. But the point is that a person living with dementia should not be at home alone for extended periods.

Next, putting together an emergency action plan is always a good idea. This plan may include which hospital your loved one will go to in case of an emergency, or what inpatient rehabilitation facility or skilled nursing facility they'll move to in case they need rehabilitation for a broken hip or other injury. Put the individual's health care information, such as a DNR (Do Not Resuscitate) order in an easily accessible place in the house, such as on the side of the fridge.

Putting It into Practice

Safety Do's and Don'ts

Before you decide on a move, you should ensure that a person living with dementia is safe at home. You may find this list of do's and don'ts helpful while your loved one is at home with you or with another full-time caregiver.

Do	Do Not
Place health care information in an accessible spot	Rely on notes
	Rely on promises
Unplug stove and electronics when not in use	Allow clutter to accumulate
Ensure that there is good lighting throughout the house, especially in stairwells	Place throw rugs on the floor

Guidelines for In-Home Caregivers

- Do not rely on notes.
- Do not rely on promises.
- Place health care information in an accessible spot.
- Clear clutter, especially in walkways, as clutter can pose a dangerous fall hazard.
- Pick up throw rugs. Throw rugs that aren't secured to the floor can also create a dangerous trip hazard.
- Unplug the stove and other appliances. If your loved one is never home alone, it may not be necessary to unplug all appliances. But if there are times when your loved is able to use appliances unassisted, you may want to consider keeping potentially dangerous ones unplugged. Even a microwave, if used improperly, can quickly cause a fire. Some families opt to take the knobs off gas stoves and tell loved ones with dementia that "the stove needs to be fixed before anyone uses it."
- Keep stairs well lit. If the person with dementia must use stairs, be sure they have adequate lighting and that the individual is able to use them safely.
- Install a stair chair or stair lift if stairs are unavoidable but too challenging for the person living with dementia to access safely.
- Keep cleaning liquids locked away. Although unlikely, there is a chance that your loved one with dementia could confuse something poisonous for a beverage.
- Lock any doors that you are able to lock, or look into installing locks that are difficult to use or require a special key.
- Install door chimes. For doors that you cannot leave locked, install a chime or alarm so you know if your loved one opens it while you are in another room.
- Affix removable clings for glass doors. Most everyone can tell you a story about accidentally walking into a glass door. Your loved one may not be able to tell the difference between a closed glass door and an open glass door, so it is advisable to attach window clings to the glass, which provides a visual cue that the door is closed.
- Use motion alarms near beds. If the person with dementia is known to get up a lot during the night, put a motion alarm under their bed that chimes when their feet hit the floor. The alarm should be loud enough to wake you up, alerting you that your loved one is out of bed and possibly in need of assistance.
- Add a chair to the shower. Shower chairs are imperative for both your safety and the safety of the individual living with dementia. Even a simple shower bench can allow a person to sit, get clean, and not risk a potential slippery fall.
- Install grab bars. It can be difficult to get on and off the commode with no grab bars. Some grab bars are attached to the wall, or you can purchase an inexpensive, adjustable toilet seat with grab bars from most medical device companies.
- Add handrailings where necessary. If there is a spot in the house where your loved one has a tendency to fall or struggle, look into getting handrails installed.
- Utilize mobility devices. If walking unassisted has become a challenge, look into getting a walker or other mobility aid. I recommend speaking to an occupational or physical therapist to see what device is best for your loved one.

What special considerations do you need to consider about your loved one's home?

_____

_____

_____

RESOURCES

National Institute on Aging. 2017. Home Safety and Alzheimer's Disease. https://www.nia.nih.gov/health/home-safety-and-alzheimers-disease.

National Institute on Aging. 2017. Home Safety Checklist for Alzheimer's Disease. https://www.nia.nih.gov/health/home-safety-checklist-alzheimers-disease.

CHAPTER 19

When Is It Time to Move Your Loved One?

Making a difficult decision a little easier

Moving your loved into a dementia care community will be a big change for you and your family, so make sure you are doing it for the right reasons—and at the right time. Perhaps you are struggling with your family member's twenty-four-hour needs. The physical and emotional demands of caregiving are weighing on you and your own independence. You may discover that a care community is the right choice. Let's review some reasons why you may need to make this big change.

Physical Needs

As a person's dementia progresses, their family may become unable to care for them physically. This is one of the most common reasons for transitioning a loved one to a dementia care community. When your parent, partner, child, or friend living with dementia requires assistance to walk, eat, and bathe, their needs can become overwhelming. You should not strain your body attempting to move or transfer them. In a dementia care community, the staff can work together—and often do—to assist residents.

Incontinence is also an issue for individuals living with moderate to advanced dementia. Urinary or bowel incontinence means that a person loses control over their bladder and bowel functions. People with dementia will eventually require disposable adult briefs made for incontinence and need frequent changing. Incontinence can be incredibly challenging—and potentially embarrassing—for family caregivers to handle. Trained, experienced staff members at dementia care communities have experience coping with incontinence in their residents and are comfortable performing this task.

Emotional Needs

Families may consider dementia care communities when they feel unable emotionally to continue caring for a parent, partner, or child living with dementia. Caring for another person is incredibly challenging and stressful. As we discussed in chapter 14, care partners have lives to live, too, and other responsibilities. Caring for a loved one living with dementia is a full-time (and usually an unpaid) job, and many caregivers *already* have a full-time job. There are instances when a family caregiver can be paid, but it depends on the state in which the family lives.

When your loved one joins a care community, you are not neglecting them; in fact, the move may even improve your relationship. Consider this: when you're constantly caring for your father, you get caught up in the stressful, day-to-day tasks and physical needs that he requires. Commonly, family caregivers lament how physically exhausting the hands-on care can become. When you visit your father in a dementia care community, the full-time staff have already met his physical needs. You are able to provide emotional support for him without worrying about the hands-on care. You are less stressed. Likely, your loved one is less stressed, too, so you two can focus on enjoying each other's company.

Safety Concerns

One of the major reasons for transitioning a family member or friend to a dementia care community is because that person is unsafe where they are living currently. Families often have trouble ensuring the safety of someone living with dementia, especially when that person lives at home. In the early stages of dementia, people can get lost in familiar places. Some people in the later stages of dementia will pace constantly, picking up objects on the way that seem interesting to them. People in the later stages often cannot verbalize who they are or where they live. If they get lost outside of the home, they may not be able to ask for help. If a person living with dementia lives at home, it may be necessary to lock the doors so that they cannot exit without the aid of a caregiver. Some companies sell door locks made specifically for this situation.

Even with an in-home care agency, your house may not be the best place for your loved one living with dementia. Floor mats or rugs can be slip hazards, negotiating stairs can result in dangerous falls, and appliances such as the stove or toaster oven can be hazardous. Although your family member or friend may feel as though they can do everything they always did, you know this isn't the case. Your mother once enjoyed baking cookies by herself, but she may now forget she left the oven on. As "dementia-proof" as you make your house, it will never be as safe as a community designed for people with cognitive loss.

When It Is Time to Join a Dementia Care Community

Perhaps your family member or friend is living in an independent living or assisted living community that is not built for people living with cognitive impairments. Recall that these communities typically don't keep the doors locked twenty-four hours a day. Residents living with dementia may not only be unsafe in one of these communities, but they may also withdraw socially. Whether your parent, partner, child, or friend lives at home alone or in a community surrounded by people, it is possible that they will lose the capacity to engage with others who are not on the same cognitive level. Some people living with dementia start withdrawing socially because they become aware of their limitations and feel embarrassed. Others withdraw out of necessity; perhaps the types of activities and programs available make no sense to them.

Unfortunately, some people in these communities, whether out of fear or cruelty, may tease or socially isolate a person living with dementia. In situations like these, it may be best to consider joining a dementia care community. Most residents in dementia care communities enjoy each other's company. They also have the opportunity to participate in easy-to-complete activities designed specifically for their needs. For example, while one resident works on a puzzle, another may sort and fold socks, while still another could arrange flowers or type on a community computer.

"Mom wants to live at home, where she has always lived," Sally said. "She loves it here; it just wouldn't be fair to relocate her." Sally spent a lot of time searching the Internet for potential caregivers. In fact, she hired three shifts of caregivers, seven days a week.

I spent two nights each week looking after Sally's 90-year-old mother, Margaret. Margaret, living in a moderate stage of Alzheimer disease, would wake up frequently throughout the night to use the bathroom. I slept in Margaret's quiet old house and woke up regularly to the sound of a motion alarm, signaling that she had gotten out of bed. I would help Margaret walk to the bathroom, use the toilet, and then get back to bed.

The more time I spent with Margaret, the more I realized that Sally was incorrect about her mother's feelings toward the house. In truth, Margaret had no idea that she still lived at home. "I had better call my husband," she would tell me. "I need to let him know that I'm staying at this hotel tonight."

———————

Margaret didn't realize that it was her house because the people she loved no longer lived there. A house is not a home unless it contains things that connect a person to it emotionally, and for Margaret, those things were not there. Margaret's husband had passed away, and her children were adults. Still, Margaret's family remained convinced that it would be cruel to move her into a dementia care community, even as they struggled to find caregivers to look after her around the clock. She often asked to "go home" even though she had lived in the house for more than fifty years. In truth, Margaret was a perfect candidate for a dementia care community and would never have realized that she was living in one.

When It's *Not* Time for a Dementia Care Community

The decision to take your parent, partner, child, or sibling to a dementia care community is a personal one. As you weigh your decision, note that there are some instances when your family member living with dementia will *not* be a good fit for a dementia care community.

Should My Loved One Be in a Non-Dementia-Care Community?

Charlie joined a dementia care community well before he was ready for the level of care it provided. His dementia symptoms were mild, and he was not ready to live in a secured community twenty-four hours a day. Charlie stayed in his room constantly. He refused to engage in any programs because he was afraid of the other residents.

"I'm sorry," he said. "I'm just afraid to talk to anyone here. Sometimes a woman walks in my room and just starts going on and on about things I don't understand. Why is she acting like that?" Although he wanted to make new friends, he was unable to find anyone at his cognitive level. Whereas other residents happily engaged with one another, Charlie was an outcast. Eventually, Charlie moved into an independent living community.

———————

Most residents living in dementia care communities adjust well to their new homes and benefit from positively interacting with others. And for the most part, even the higher-functioning residents do not realize that there is anything abnormal about others who live in the community. But when a resident is frightened of other people in the community or believes they are "crazy," they are *not* a good fit for a dementia-specific unit.

A doctor may occasionally suggest dementia community placement for a person who isn't yet ready for it. Overall, you need to know your family member's level of dementia to decide whether a dementia care community is appropriate. Recognize that some communities will have higher-functioning residents than others and may offer different levels of activities. Visit your local dementia-specific communities to decide what is best for your parent, partner, child, or sibling. You'll know almost immediately if there are residents at the community with whom they will be able to interact.

Should My Loved One Be in a Skilled Nursing Facility?

Your family member may require more care than a dementia care community typically provides. They might be better off in a skilled nursing facility. Nursing facilities are typically for residents who require complete, or nearly complete, physical assistance. For example, if your mother uses a wheelchair, needs to be fed, cannot be transferred to a bed or a toilet without assistance from at least two people, and is completely incontinent, she may be a good fit for a nursing facility. Sadly, some family members wait too long to choose a dementia care community. By the time they decide on one, the person with dementia is a better candidate for a nursing home.

When deciding whether a dementia care community is right for your mother, for example, ask yourself these important questions.

1. Is your mother able to interact with others? Will she be able to make friends at a dementia care community?
2. Is mom more of an introvert? Would she do better with one-on-one care or with larger groups?
3. Have you talked to the nurse or director at your local dementia-specific community? They may be able to tell you if the community has other residents with the same physical needs as your mother.
4. Will your mother enjoy participating group activities or performances?
5. What are the costs associated with each community? Is a dementia care community more expensive?
6. Will your mother get enough positive interaction from a nursing home? Although cost is important, it's also necessary to weigh the benefits your mother will get from living in a more connected community.
7. What are the policies about visiting hours? You want to make sure that you can check in on your loved one and bring other members of the family to visit. Have things changed since the COVID-19 pandemic? Are the rules likely to change again?

If your mother would have a better life at a dementia-specific community, you should choose that as her new home. Visit a few communities if possible, to get a feel for the environment they provide. If you can't visit in person, you may be able to take a virtual tour online (Memory Center). Above all, trust your gut feeling. And when it comes to a disaster or change in visiting rules, what is the plan? What happened to the community during the peak of the pandemic, and what has changed since then?

Wherever you choose to move your parent, partner, child, or sibling, don't get discouraged if they don't immediately fit in. Even though they may ask to go home or complain about other residents, give them time to get used to the community. It is important for family members to recognize that many residents take time to fully adjust to a new environment.

Putting It into Practice

The goal of this exercise is to help you decide if moving someone to a care community is the right thing to do. Recall the phrase "If you're thinking about it, it's probably time." In the next few chapters, we will review other steps of the decision-making process. Below are the steps that I generally recommend when deciding to move someone, choosing a place, and then making the transition.

1. Decide if you need to move someone living with dementia to another setting, such as a care community. This step involves doing some self-reflection, knowing the individual who will be moving, seeking out information (like reading this book), and asking friends and family for advice. Take account of the following:

Cognitive needs of your loved one:

_____

Physical needs of your loved one:

_____

Emotional needs of your loved one:

_____

Your physical needs:

_____

Your emotional needs:

_____

Safety concerns:

_____

Location needs (How far away do you live? Who is able to visit?):

_____

2. Go on Google Maps or an equivalent program and determine the area in which this person would be living. Choosing a care community is an overwhelming decision, and location is one of the most important pieces of this process. The location will also help inform your decision to move them. Are there any facilities close to where they currently live or near where you currently live? Will friends and family be likely and able to visit?

3. Search for the type of community that you are interested in on the maps program. In the next chapter, we will go into the different types of communities.

4. Visit communities by yourself, with a friend or family member, or even with the person you are considering moving.

5. Once you've chosen a community, fill out any required paperwork, ask questions, and solve any potential issues with the marketing director and administrators ahead of time. The last thing you want to be is stressed and unprepared the day of the actual move. See chapter 23, "Move-In Day," for more on the logistics of making the move.

RESOURCES

National Institute on Aging. 2017. Finding Long-Term Care for a Person with Alzheimer's. https://www.nia.nih.gov/health/finding-long-term-care-person-alzheimers.

The Memory Center. 2016. Virtual Tour. https://www.thememorycenter.com/virtual-tour-2/.

CHAPTER 20

What Types of Communities Exist?

Similarities and differences among care communities

Decades ago, if a loved one showed signs of being "senile," there wasn't much to be done. Most people with symptoms of cognitive loss lived and died at home or went to nursing facilities. Personally, I think this is part of the reason that people are so afraid of the idea of a nursing home and often tell their loved ones something along the lines of, "Don't ever move me to a home!" These days, we don't even use the words "senile" and "senility"—when people used those words, they were actually describing dementia. There is a stereotype about what dementia care is and what it looks like, and most of it is based on outdated information, stereotypes in movies and on television, and fear. Often, when people think of "a home," they think of old folks sitting in wheelchairs, staring out steel-barred windows in smelly, hospital-like hallways.

Care partners tell me they fear that their only two choices are to "keep their loved one at home or move them to long-time care." In reality, there are a number of lifestyle options for older adults with cognitive impairments. As we review these options, remember that each one has pros and cons. Bear in mind that senior living options will vary from location to location and country to country, so what you read here may not reflect all the options in your area. In addition, some states have different names for the same or similar type of care in another state. I've heard options like "supported living" or "adult foster care" in some areas of the United States. My best advice is to keep an open mind and learn as much as you can about the options available to you and your family.

Independent Living Communities

Independent living (IL) communities for seniors are places where residents are offered meals, activities, and outings but are free to go about their day as they see fit. Residents of IL communities live independently. We can best liken this type of community to a college environment: there are things to do, but technically you do not have to leave your room if you don't want to. Most IL communities offer apartment-style living: each unit has a kitchenette, a bathroom, a bedroom or two, and a living room. Some units come fully furnished, while others only offer a bed and appliances. Although there are plenty of older adults with cognitive impairments who live in IL communities, I do not recommend moving someone living with a dementia diagnosis to one. People living with dementia are eventually unable to live independently, so moving someone with dementia to an IL community means that they'll either struggle to receive care or that you will have to move them again before too long.

One option is for a care partner and the person they are caring to move to an IL community together. The care partner has some reprieve, as they don't have to take care of cleaning a house and mowing a lawn, and they are able to focus on caregiving. Independent living communities tend to be less expensive because the staff does not provide hands-on care compared to other senior living options.

Assisted Living Communities and Personal Care Homes

If we are likening independent living to college, we can liken assisted living facilities (ALFs) or personal care homes (PCHs) to a high-school-type environment. In contrast with IL communities, there is more supervision in ALFs for individuals that need it, although there is still a good deal of freedom. There are activities and meals, and staff ensure that residents are reminded about programs and dining on a regular basis. While some residents still drive and park their vehicles at the community, most do not, and instead rely on community transportation. Residents are usually required to sign in and out when leaving the building.

Many ALFs and PCHs have memory care hallways, although some communities use a different term. Memory care (here identified as dementia care) is a side of the building, a hallway, a wing, or unit that is designated for people living with dementia. The first ALF that I worked in had an entirely different building for residents living with dementia, called the Reminiscence Unit. Sometimes what families will do is move a loved one with earlier stages of cognitive loss into the AL side of the building, and then transition them to the dementia care side when it becomes necessary.

Dementia Care Communities

I am giving dementia care communities (DCCs) their own section because the needs of adults with cognitive decline differ from those of healthy adults. More and more companies are establishing new facilities to meet the needs of people living with dementia. Although these facilities carry licenses for assisted living or personal care, they only cater to adults with dementia.

Depending on their management and location, dementia care communities are often secure, and residents cannot leave the community without assistance. This may seem intimidating at first, but it's for the residents' safety. People living with dementia sometimes attempt to "go home" or "go outside" and end up getting lost. Residents are able to go outside the community when a friend, family member, or staff member accompanies them. Some communities also have a center courtyard where residents can come and go as they please.

Dementia care communities are staffed twenty-four hours a day, seven days a week. Usually, three shifts of employees and staff members care for residents around the clock. Administrative staff are only on-site during normal business hours, so if you have an important question, try to find someone on your family member or friend's management team between the hours of 9:00 a.m. and 5:00 p.m.

When considering a DCC, be sure to visit and ensure the organization running the community knows and understands positive dementia care. Unfortunately, some companies that create DCCs have no prior interest or knowledge in dementia care. Let me repeat my warning to you: *Be sure that the organization running the community knows and understands positive dementia care.*

Sometimes, a group such as an architectural firm will set out to create a dementia-specific building but lack understanding for the type of care that happens there. Dementia care buildings are in high demand, and where there is a business need, a company is ready to pop up and fill it.

I have been introduced to plenty of brand-new organizations full of lovely people who want to make DCCs a happier, safer place to live. For example, a new organization in Tennessee contacted me to train their core staff on dementia care techniques. Remember Me Senior Care was established because a family who lost their mother to Alzheimer disease was displeased with the care options available to her in life. They set out to create a senior living community that was catered to older adults living with dementia, armed with the right goals and knowledge. Wherever and whatever the community, be sure to find out who owns the building and *why* they own it.

Nursing Homes

Nursing homes are facilities that families often reference when they feel as though they must move a loved one. Within a nursing home there are two levels of care: skilled nursing—a skilled nursing facility is often referred to as an SNF—and long-term care. An SNF is a specific licensure, different from assisted living, and run by a nursing home administrator. The rules and regulations in SNFs are much stricter than those of an assisted living building or other care community, so the person running the SNF must have a nursing home administrator's license. The knowledge required to pass the SNF licensure exam is far greater than to pass the exam to be the executive director of an ALF.

Anyone can go to an SNF, including, for example, a young person who needs rehabilitation and physical therapy following a serious injury. Residents who qualify to stay at an SNF are usually there for short-term rehabilitation or require skilled nursing care. Because the residents of an SNF require medical care and/or physical assistance, it makes sense that SNF staff are medically trained. Among the people who work in SNFs are trained certified nursing assistants (CNAs), licensed practical nurses (LPNs), and registered nurses (RNs).

Because of the increased level of care an individual receives in an SNF, services cost more than care in other types of communities. So, residents at an SNF will receive help from their Medicare insurance plan. Once their Medicare days have been exhausted, they no longer have a skilled need, or if they have received up to one hundred days of skilled care within a year's time, they can convert to Medicaid if they financially qualify or pay out of pocket. (The cost of care is covered more thoroughly in chapter 18.)

Nursing homes also have long-term care units, which is often where their residents with cognitive impairments live. Not every nursing home has a dementia-specific wing or hallway, so it's important to ask about this before moving a loved one living with dementia into a nursing home.

Respite Care

Most assisted living facilities offer "respite stays," usually short stays for a minimum of ten days. Respite care is an option for families who are considering moving a loved one but may not be ready yet. It is also an option for families who are going away on vacation or working on a big home project and thus need care for a loved one living with dementia who can't be at home alone.

Communities that offer respite stays are hoping to convert short-term prospects into long-term residents. They're hoping that your family likes the community so much that you fill out the paperwork to move your loved one there as a full-time resident.

Most communities will ask you to complete all the required paperwork to become a full-time resident even if it's only a ten-day stay. You can't just show up with a loved one, drop them off, and go on your trip. Frankly, even if you could do this, it would not be advisable, because transitions take time and patience. Respite stay move-ins should be treated with the same care and consideration as permanent move-ins. Although respite stays provide coverage for you and give you and your loved one a firsthand experience in a particular care community, there are downsides. Because they are relatively short stays, it can be difficult for your loved one with dementia to feel comfortable in their temporary home. It is also difficult for staff to develop the relationships needed to best help your loved one. While working in different assisted living communities, I would meet a new resident on a respite stay, begin to get to know them, and then their family would move them out.

Continuing Care Retirement Communities

Continuing care retirement communities (CCRCs) provide multiple levels of care, such as independent living, assisted living, personal care, skilled nursing, and long-term care. The expectation is that many residents will move from one type of care to another as needed. For example, your family member or friend could move into independent living at a CCRC, and then later move to assisted living, and then into a dementia care community. One great thing about CCRCs is that your aging parent, partner, or friend is typically guaranteed a spot in the next level of community care. If you suspect that they will need multiple levels of care, consider a CCRC as you visit various communities.

Home Care Agencies

Home care agencies are companies that will send a caregiver to provide care in your loved one's home. Home care agencies can send caregivers into senior living communities, too, so these services are not relegated to just home care. A family may consider hiring a home care agency to provide extra one-to-one care for their loved one in a long-term care community. Note, however, that if your loved one is not receiving the right care in their community, it may make more sense to move them to a different place rather than spend money for additional outside assistance. The benefit of home care agencies is that if a scheduled caregiver is unable to be there, the agency is supposed to send someone in their place.

Home care agencies are sometimes mom-and-pop shops, individually or family owned small businesses. More often, however, home care agencies are franchises. The biggest in the United States is Home Instead Senior Care. Franchise owners run their local business but receive marketing materials, guidelines, training, and other information from the parent company. Choosing a franchise over a small business is a personal decision, and how good the company is depends on the people in the office and the caregivers they hire and train.

Most home care agencies have minimums for the number of hours of care that they will provide each week. Some have two or three three-hour shift minimums, which could make it difficult if you only want help once a week. Most of these agencies charge by the hour, sometimes offering discounts to low-income clients or veterans. Bear in mind that there are two types of home care agencies: medical and nonmedical. Most home care agencies, such as Home Instead Senior Care, are nonmedical. Depending on state regulations, nonmedical care agencies cannot give medication to a client; they can only monitor that someone takes their medication. Medical care agencies are staffed by trained nurses and provide more physical care, such as Foley catheter care. Talk with your local home care agency about what they can and cannot provide before signing up for care.

Adult Day Care

A dult day care is what it sounds like: daytime care for older adults— usually people living with dementia. Many adult day care communities are open from the morning hours until early evening. Adult day care communities offer a variety of programs and activities, but they are typically designed for people who don't have significant physical care needs. For example, someone who is completely incontinent and requires a shower after a bathroom accident is not a great fit for adult day care.

Adult day care is a great option for families who are looking to eventually move a loved one living with dementia into a full-time care community but aren't ready to complete the move just yet. Among all the assisted living and personal care communities out there, adult day communities are the least common. Many families aren't aware that adult day care is even an option. To find an adult day care near you, check out your state's official government website. For example, in Pennsylvania, where I live, you can find more information about adult day care by county and even check when the facility was last inspected: https://www.aging.pa.gov /local-resources/Pages/Adult-Day -Center.aspx.

Choosing the Right Community

Choosing the right community at the right time for your loved one with dementia is a real art form. I have had residents move into assisted living who were much more appropriate for long-term nursing care. It is unlikely that someone will move "too soon"; it is much more likely that a family will wait too long. The only way to know for sure whether a community is a good fit is to speak to the people who work at the community. A nurse or social worker from the building will come to evaluate your loved one. They will, hopefully, in their best judgment, be able to tell you if your loved one fits in their level of care.

Make every effort to visit the community twice before making a decision. Try going at different times of day and on different days, and be aware that residents usually grow more agitated later in the afternoon, as they may be sundowning.

Talk with residents' family members to get a good feel for the community. Ask others about their experiences, and learn what they like and dislike about the community. You can also learn much by watching staff interact with the residents.

Putting It into Practice

Check your bias: When you hear "nursing home," what comes to mind?

Look back through your answers to the Putting It into Practice questions in chapter 19. Do you believe that it's time, or will soon be time, to move your loved one? Based on your answers and the reading of this chapter, what is your first, gut instinct as to which type of community might be best?

Your family member or friend living with dementia may need a type of care that differs from what someone else needs. For some families, in-home care works best, but for others, dementia care communities are better options. As long as you are providing your family member or friend with the best physical and emotional care you can manage, you are doing the right thing. Don't let anyone make you feel as if you have taken the "easy way out" by choosing a dementia care community. You still have to cope with a lot of challenging behaviors, emotions, and concerns when it comes to your family member's care.

Here is a list of questions to ask when looking for a care community. Bear in mind that many of these can be learned through observation, rather than asking someone directly:

- Does the community host family gatherings or support groups?
- What does the community look like? Are there common areas that will provide comfort to your parent, friend, or partner? For example, some communities have a "baby station" with realistic-looking baby dolls, bottles, and baby clothes. Many residents love cuddling and talking to the dolls.
- Are there safe areas where the residents can sit outdoors while remaining within the walls of the community?
- Do the people who work there seem helpful and kind?
- Do the staff members seem to really know and care about each resident?
- Do they attend to residents quickly and with familiarity?
- When the staff speak to residents, do they talk at them or with them?
- How do the other residents look? Do they look well groomed and healthy? Are any of them close to your friend or family member's level of need? For example, you would not want to move your mother living with mild dementia into a community where the other residents are more progressed in dementia and cannot speak or engage with her.

CHAPTER 21

Cost of Care

How much does dementia care cost?

Notes on the Cost of Dementia Care

In this chapter, I review costs associated with caring for people living with dementia. Although I provide an overview of these costs, specific charges vary from place to place. Medicare and Medicaid information changes as well, so be sure to obtain the most up-to-date information on Medicare and Medicaid from your local area agency on aging or from an elder law expert.

The cost for dementia care is high. This isn't just the cost for the family or individual of the person living with dementia; the cost of dementia care for society in general is high. Consider the tasks of a woman who is caring for her father, who is living with dementia. She probably has a career and perhaps a family at home. As her father's dementia progresses, she must begin to provide extra care for him. She loses wages as she takes more time off from work, and her employer begins to feel the strain, albeit on a different scale, as they lose money and time a successful employee once provided. Unpaid caregivers are

predominately women, who are juggling their own lives in addition to the life of the person living with dementia. On average, these caregivers provide twenty hours of unpaid labor each week— equivalent to a part-time job.

Now, consider that this woman wants to get some extra help caring for her father. Does she decide to bring in a home care agency? Try adult day care? Perhaps move him into a dementia care community? How does she know what each will cost, or how to pay for the care? Although the actual cost varies by country and by city, the overall impact of dementia caregiving is immense. In this chapter, I break down the types of care and how they are paid for, along with some potential costs that you may encounter during your own caregiving journey.

Where you live will play a major role in the financial cost of a senior living community. Some states, cities, and counties have programs that help people pay for senior living, and I always advise curious family members to do their homework before making a big financial change. For example, the state of Minnesota offers an elderly waiver or alternative care program that can help families pay for senior care. I personally had no idea this existed before I visited Minnesota for a consulting job, and it got me thinking: What else do people not know about when it comes to paying for elder care? If you are worried that you'll have to downsize or sell your home, please be sure to do your research, and consider speaking with an elder law attorney before making a big decision. The American Bar Association has a dedicated page on its website about finding a specialist lawyer in your state. There's a chance that the outlook of your situation is more positive than you've previously assumed. Good elder law attorneys know the ins and outs of financial and legal decisions in senior caregiving in your local area.

Types of Care

Dementia care is, without a doubt, more expensive than the rest of aging care. In the area where I live (Pittsburgh, Pennsylvania), we have a large population of older adults and many senior care facilities. I always ask about the cost of care at communities I visit and have found that dementia care is, on average, $2,000 more a month than non-dementia-specific assisted living care. Assisted living in this area begins around $4,500 a month, and when you add dementia care, prices can get into the $6,500 range. If you think that home care would be a better option for your loved one, consider that most home care agencies charge $22 to $25 an hour, at least in the Pittsburgh area.

Dementia care communities should include more hands-on care than other care communities. They should have secured doors, dementia-friendly activities, and socialization with others who are living with dementia. Although they are more expensive, these benefits make them better options for someone living with dementia. In many of these communities, different rooms have different costs. For example, a large private room is going to be more expensive than a small or shared double room. A room with a better view could be slightly more expensive than a room without much of a view. Recently, I've noticed that more communities are opting for all-inclusive pricing, a policy that I think makes sense. An all-inclusive fee means that even if your loved one's needs change, their cost of care would remain the same.

In North Carolina, I worked at a community where we had a few residents on Medicaid. Pennsylvania, on the other hand, does not currently accept residents into assisted living or personal care using Medicaid assistance as a means to pay. In some communities, care partners need to demonstrate the ability to pay for at least the first couple years of care. Long-term care insurance can help individuals who had purchased it before they needed care.

The take-home message is, the earlier a person begins planning financially for elder care, the better.

As I mentioned in chapter 20, independent living communities are not good places for people living with dementia. Unfortunately, I have seen families keep a person living with dementia in independent living for much longer than they should to save money, as independent living is generally much cheaper than other types of care. But this is why it's called "independent" living. There are no care costs included because residents are assumed to be independent.

Long-term care facilities or nursing homes are significantly more expensive than assisted living or dementia care communities, but they generally accept Medicaid. For many families, nursing homes are a last resort because of their hospital-like appearance and feel. For a loved one with substantial physical needs or financial concerns, nursing homes are an important option.

Health insurance might pay for a person's occupational therapy, speech therapy, or physical therapy if they require these services. Nursing homes and often assisted living facilities with dementia care communities have their own therapy team available on-site. Therapy providers visit patients in their rooms or meet them in a therapy suite.

Breakdown of Costs

Good hygiene is an important part of life, especially for people living with dementia. Although an adult with a diagnosis of dementia could once dress herself, toilet independently, and eat without assistance, as her disease progresses, she is left with less and less ability to care for her own activities of daily living (ADLs). She now requires the help of others when it comes to cleanliness and hygiene. In a dementia care community, assistance with ADLs comes with a large price tag.

The fee structure varies among care communities. For example, some bill separate room charges and care charges. When choosing a care community for your parent, partner, child, or friend, research in advance what charges will appear on each bill. Is the community's care all-inclusive? Will costs go up as a resident progresses in their disease? Most likely, you'll see a base charge for rent in addition to charges for a resident's care and care products. In many communities, as a person's care needs increase, these care charges grow and are added to a family's bill each month.

"We were never told about this charge," the woman said angrily. "Our aunt wasn't supposed to be charged this much for care! Why are we paying for someone to take her to the bathroom? She is able to do that herself!"

Sophia's family was angry, and they had a right to be. They had a hard time understanding why they were paying more now, especially when Sophia had, according to them, been toileting herself independently for years. Now, as Sophia's disease progressed, her care charges increased. On top of her rent for the room, the community now charged Sophia's family for an aide's time to help her use the bathroom each day. Her cost had gone up significantly as her condition had worsened. Although frustrating, increasing costs over time are common at senior care communities.

"We were only told about the rent base rate," they argued. "We thought it stopped there!"

Find out what is included in a community's price tag before making the move, and get the answers in writing. For example, ask if residents' toilet paper, wipes, briefs, or staff gloves are included in the cost. Some communities charge separately for briefs, wipes, and gloves, all of which are used by staff when providing personal care to residents. The more details you know up front about the cost of being a resident, the fewer headaches you will have later.

Medicare and Medicaid

*M*edicare is a US federal program for adults 65 years of age and older, people under the age of 65 who receive Social Security disability benefits, and those with either amyotrophic lateral sclerosis (ALS), also called Lou Gehrig's disease, or end-stage renal disease. What long-term care services Medicare pays for can be confusing to understand.

Medicaid is a joint state and federal program that assists individuals with limited means who are living below the poverty level. Medicaid programs vary from state to state, but it's important not to rule out Medicaid as an option for nursing home care, even if the person did not previously qualify for Medicaid. Most of the individuals who utilize Medicaid fall within our two most vulnerable populations: older adults and children.

When Does Medicare Pay for a Skilled Nursing Facility?
Following Hospitalization
Medicare will help pay for a short stay in a skilled nursing facility (SNF) if you meet all of the following conditions:

- You have had a *hospital admission* with an inpatient stay of at least *three days*.
- You are admitted to a *Medicare-certified nursing facility within 30 days* of that inpatient hospital stay.
- You need *skilled care*, such as skilled nursing services, occupational therapy, physical therapy and/or speech therapy.

If you meet all these conditions, Medicare will pay a portion of the costs for up to *one hundred days* for each benefit period as follows:

- For the *first twenty days, Medicare pays 100%* of the cost.

- For *days twenty-one through one hundred, you pay a daily copayment, which was $164.50* as of November 2017), and Medicare pays any balance.
- Medicare does not pay costs for days you stay in a skilled nursing facility after one hundred days.

To Treat Medical Conditions

Medicare pays for the following services when your doctor prescribes them as medically necessary to treat an illness or injury:

- Part-time or intermittent skilled nursing care.
- Physical therapy, occupational therapy, and speech-language pathology provided by a *Medicare-certified* home health agency.
- Medical social services to help cope with the social, psychological, cultural, and medical issues that result from an illness. This may include help accessing services and follow-up care, explaining how to use health care and other resources, and help understanding your disease.
- Medical supplies and durable medical equipment such as wheelchairs, hospital beds, oxygen, and walkers. For durable medical equipment, Medicare pays 80% of the approved amount, and you pay 20%.

To Prevent Further Decline Due to Medical Conditions

In some cases, Medicare also covers ongoing long-term care services to prevent further decline for people with medical conditions that may not improve. This coverage can include conditions like stroke, Parkinson's disease, ALS, multiple sclerosis, or Alzheimer disease.

Points to Take Away

My best advice is this: don't panic when thinking about the cost of caring for someone living with dementia. I know it feels impossible and overwhelming, but the first and most important thing to do is consider what your loved one living with dementia needs. What kind of care do they really need? What kind of care would they want, had they been able to make this choice for themselves? What do you want for them, or what do you think is best? Throughout the rest of this book, we will work to uncover answers to challenging questions like these. Consider talking to an elder law attorney, even if that just means a quick question-and-answer phone call. There are also a variety of placement agencies out there that will help families decide where to transition a loved one. Bear in mind that these types of businesses receive referral monies from senior living organizations, although they are free to the consumer.

Putting It into Practice

Questions to ask a care community about cost:

1. What is included in this price?
2. Are wipes, gloves, adult briefs, and other supplies included?
3. What happens if my loved one declines? Is the extra care included, or will the cost of their care go up? If so, by how much?
4. Is there a sliding scale for fees based on income or assets?
5. What programs are available to someone if they run out of money?
6. What happens if they run out of money while they live here?

RESOURCES

Administration for Community Living. 2021. What Is Long-Term Care (LTC) and Who Needs It? https://longtermcare.acl.gov/.

Alzheimer's Association. 2020. Planning Ahead for Long-Term Care Expenses. https://www.alz.org/media/documents/alzheimers-dementia-plan-ahead-long-term-care-expenses-ts.pdf.

American Bar Association. Bar Directories and Lawyer Finders. 2021. https://www.americanbar.org/groups/legal_services/flh-home/flh-bar-directories-and-lawyer-finders/.

Medicare.gov. 2021. How Can I Pay for Nursing Home Care? https://www.medicare.gov/what-medicare-covers/what-part-a-covers/how-can-i-pay-for-nursing-home-care.

PART IV

Caregiving in a Care Community

What about when a loved one finally transitions to a care community? What if they're already living there? In this section, I talk about care within a care community setting and why caregiving is an imperfect science. I discuss day trips and outings, activities and programming, along with what dementia-friendly interior design really means.

CHAPTER 22

What to Expect at a Dementia Care Community

Things to know and things to ask about

In this chapter, we explore what you should expect regarding direct care in a dementia care community. By direct care, I am referring to bathing, toileting, dressing, eating, keeping up with oral care, and doing laundry. Care will differ depending on the type of community you choose. For example, in most *independent living community environments*, the community does *not* provide assistance for residents in the shower or give reminders about mealtimes—good reasons not to choose this type of environment for someone living with dementia. In *assisted living environments not specifically designed for people with dementia*, some physical care is provided by staff members, but the staff will likely operate under the assumption that residents are able to complete their activities of daily living (ADLs) without much extra assistance. "Activities of daily living" is a term that you will hear come up often in conversations about caregiving. It is used to describe such activities as eating, bathing, getting dressed, being able to get around (mobility), and controlling

bladder and bowel functions. Any additional hands-on care usually will be available for an extra fee. Designated *dementia care communities* are the only ones that cater directly to the special needs of those living with dementia.

I often speak to caregivers who express exhaustion over their friend or family member's increasing physical and cognitive care needs. Just recently, a man emailed me about his wife, whom he was caring for at home. They were both in their late 80s and struggling, with no nearby family to help. "She won't get in the shower, and even if she did, I fear she's at risk for a fall," he explained in his email. "She now needs me to change her regularly throughout the day, and it's a lot of physical work for me. I have a bad back, and I find myself truly tired at the end of the day! I feel guilty, but I'm so glad when she finally falls asleep—I get a small reprieve."

Families may feel guilty when they aren't able to provide constant, ongoing physical and cognitive care to a person living with dementia. But then, they wonder, *Would moving them to a dementia care community be any better? What could the community provide that they couldn't?*

The simplest answer is that dementia care communities have round-the-clock staff members who are trained to provide dementia care. Yes, the staff is providing more care to more people, but new staff comes in every eight hours or so. This is the opposite of caring for someone at home, where it's just that one care partner, each day, every day, around the clock. Of course, there are not-so-great communities out there. I sometimes hear people say, "Well, I moved my mom to so-and-so, and it was awful. I'm never trying another place!" I advise these families that, while I believe they did have a bad experience, not every community is the same. There's a great chance that another community would be a better fit.

Personal History

When joining a dementia care community, you will be asked to complete a document with details about the resident's personal history. The form typically includes details about what name or nickname the resident likes to be called, favorite pastimes, treasured possessions, regular habits and routines, preferred ways to communicate, and anything else that may be important for making a resident feel at home. These details are then shared with appropriate staff members so that everyone has the same information. Let's look at some specific direct care performed at dementia care communities along with some important details to keep in mind when evaluating facilities.

Bathing

Dementia care communities vary in their bathroom setups. Some communities have communal showers, whereas others place showers in the residents' rooms. There is no one "right" layout for a dementia community's bathrooms, so long as residents are safe while using them. Care aides at the community help residents take showers or baths, depending on the resident's preference.

The personal history form will have questions specifically related to bathing preferences, so it's important to provide as much detail as possible. Imagine, for example, if you were someone who always took a shower in the morning. Now, suddenly, care staff is helping you take a bath at night. Would this throw off your daily rhythm? Of course it would!

Most communities provide showers or baths for each resident twice a week.

If your loved one loves to bathe and wants to get a shower more often, that is probably something you can arrange—potentially for an additional fee—at the community. Otherwise, twice a week is considered normal for older adults in these settings, particularly those who are not doing strenuous exercise.

Find out if you need to supply towels, shampoo, and soaps before moving your loved one into a care community. Some places will provide towels but not soap or shampoo. It is imperative that families know what types of products are allowed at their chosen dementia care community. Different states and countries have different regulations about the types of products they allow residents to have. Although it may seem bizarre that communities would take products away from residents, it's only for safety's sake. For example, a resident could confuse a shampoo left on a countertop for a beverage. If that resident drinks the shampoo, they could get very sick—or even die. No care community wants that to happen, so many places have specific regulations about what products they allow. Most communities allow any shampoos or soaps so long as they are kept under lock and key. Residents with more mild stages of dementia can find this type of security frustrating.

It takes a lot of patience and understanding from family caregivers and care aides alike to provide residents with the best possible hygiene care. Although a person living with dementia won't lose the ability overnight to care for himself, as the disease progresses, he will need more hands-on care over time.

Toileting

Many families cite incontinence as a reason they are looking into long-term care for a loved one. Although it can be embarrassing to talk about, it's even more challenging and frustrating to handle alone. Changing a partner's adult briefs may be physically difficult, especially for an older spousal couple.

In dementia care communities, however, professional caregivers must deal with this situation constantly. Aides are often assigned specific residents by location. These aides "round" and check their residents hourly to prevent residents from soiling themselves, going to the bathroom in the wrong spot, or sitting in wet undergarments for long periods of time. Care staff members "do their changes" again before they leave for the day. Changing residents' briefs and taking residents to the restroom is arguably one of care staff members' most important tasks.

There should never be an inordinate number of residents assigned to any one caregiver—and the exact ratio required in each community varies by state and country. In my experience, more than a 1:7 ratio (one care aide responsible for seven residents) is overwhelming for care aides. *It's important to ask about the community's ratio of aides to residents* before choosing it as someone's new home. Residents living with dementia typically require more care and observation than residents without cognitive impairments, so dementia care communities should have a greater aide-to-residents ratio than other facilities.

Care communities in which residents are not checked frequently or are left in wet undergarments for too long can emit a bad odor. In some situations, communities will have to rip up and replace soiled floors to ensure it smells fresh and clean. There is no reason that a dementia care community should smell bad all the time. When searching for the right community, caregivers should look for a place that smells and looks clean—at least a majority of the time. It is important to understand, however, that there will be days when a resident has had an accident and a particular part of the community smells unpleasant. *Visit the community twice before choosing it for your parent, partner, child, or friend.* With different days come different situations, different smells, and different amounts of activity and cleanliness.

Some residents, no matter what arrangements are made for them, will struggle with the ability to use the bathroom at the right time. Take Shirley, who was notorious in one of my communities for defecating in trash cans. Shirley had a lot of trouble finding her room, so when she needed to use the bathroom, Shirley found the next best thing—a trash can, which resembled a toilet. Shirley ruined a number of trash cans before the staff devised a toileting schedule that worked for her.

Like Shirley, some residents have trouble finding the bathroom or recognizing when it is "time to go." If someone living with dementia lives long enough with the disease, that person will have trouble with incontinence. Many residents in care communities wear disposable adult briefs made specifically for people with incontinence issues. Some care communities provide briefs without charge, others provide briefs and charge for them, and still others require a resident's family to supply briefs. *It's a good idea to ask about incontinence products before choosing a specific care community.*

Oral Care

Oral hygiene often falls by the wayside for individuals living with dementia. I've seen this happen both in people's homes and in assisted living environments. It can sometimes be truly difficult to get a person living with dementia to brush their teeth. Although incredibly important—as oral hygiene is linked to overall general health—it is often overlooked.

Supply the person who is moving into a care community with their favorite type of toothbrush. Recognize that a fancy, electric toothbrush may not be a great substitute for a normal brush. If they are used to using one type of toothbrush, don't change it! As with any other items you bring for your loved one, be sure to label the toothbrush with their name or initials.

Staff should always ensure that their residents are, in the very least, using mouthwash twice a day. Many older adults have dentures, which also require special care and cleaning. If a person living with dementia refuses to brush their teeth, it could be for one or more of these reasons:

1. They forget how to use a toothbrush or misunderstand its purpose.
2. They can't see the water coming out of the faucet or are alarmed by it.
3. They don't like the feel of the brush, or perhaps have mouth sores that cause pain when brushing.

In certain cases, using mouthwash may be a substitute when a brush just won't do. For those who seem fearful of water, consider using a bowl of warm water to dip a brush into. For some people, a quick hand-over-hand use of the toothbrush—holding the hand or wrist of the other person, or having them hold your hand while you hold the brush—while brushing their teeth can work.

Dressing

I once met a family who'd purchased their mother a brand-new wardrobe before moving her into a dementia care community. While it was a loving gesture and gift from her sons, the woman had become completely overwhelmed and confused by her new clothes. Although they'd taken care to sew her name into each of her articles of clothing, it didn't help: she was convinced that none of the new clothes belonged to her. It made sense, though, because she didn't recognize the new wardrobe! Her sons had tossed out the old clothes and replaced them with new ones in the hopes that it would make her feel good and excited, but it actually just confused her even more. She spent hours crying in front of her closet when they'd visit, insisting that the "mean people working there" were hiding all her favorite sweaters.

I tell this story to illustrate a simple point: *don't fix something that isn't broken.*

If mom cycles between the same five sweaters every week, don't buy her a bunch of new tops because you want her to dress nicely at her new home. She's already in a new place; she doesn't need an entirely new (and therefore confusing) wardrobe, too.

Caregivers in home settings often report that dressing their loved ones can be frustrating. Care aides in dementia care communities will provide assistance with dressing residents, helping them with the process in a step-by-step fashion. Care aides will help residents select clothing that is comfortable and won't cause problems. For example, it's easier to wear shirts that button in the front rather than pullovers, in which a person may get stuck trying to pull it over their head. Also, a resident should have comfortable shoes that won't cause them to slip, leading to a potential fall or other injury.

Laundry

Will the care community do your loved one's laundry? How often will they wash their clothes? Is it possible for family members to do it? These are important questions to ask when choosing a care community.

Some care communities charge extra for the staff to process laundry, so some families opt to do it themselves. It's a matter of preference and cost, but I will add that it's sometimes easier to keep track of a person's clothing when the family is in charge of laundry. It is not uncommon for tops and pants to go missing in another residents' room, float around for a bit, and then, with any luck, be returned to the original wearer's room. There isn't much you can do to prevent another resident from borrowing your loved one's clothes. As I often tell care partners (and staff), this is dementia caregiving—things happen, but the things that happen aren't always worth worrying about.

Eating

It is common to walk into the dining area of a dementia care community and notice multiple residents eating completely different meals. For example, while the meal for a specific date may be chicken breast and green beans with a side of soup, you may notice various residents eating variations on that meal. One person is cutting up the chicken breast with their fork and knife, another is eating pureed chicken off a spoon, another is eating ground or pre-cut chicken, and another is being fed. We'll cover more on these dietary needs in a later chapter.

Staff members keep track of the residents' dietary needs. Even when it comes to passing out snacks, staff members should have the dietary list nearby. It's imperative, for example, that a person on a pureed diet does not accidentally get handed a plate full of food that they have to cut up and chew. As dementia progresses, individuals living with dementia may develop difficulties with chewing and swallowing. Pureed diets help prevent a resident from choking or aspirating on their food. In some communities, residents are split up by dining room table based on their dietary needs. There isn't a right or wrong way to arrange a dining room, so long as everyone's needs are met.

Once someone progresses to the point where they need to be fed, a staff member is assigned to assist them at mealtimes. It's common to see a staff member sitting with two different residents, helping to feed both of them by switching between bites. Sometimes, a resident on hospice will have the added benefit of a hospice nurse or aid who assists them directly during mealtimes.

In the next chapter, we'll talk about the details involved in moving into a dementia care community.

Putting It into Practice

Here's a list of questions to ask when researching a dementia care community:

What is the staff-to-resident ratio?

As my loved one's needs increase, what happens to their care? Who will assist them?

What do the bathrooms look like? Is there one in each room?

How are the rooms laid out? Will my loved one have their own space, or will they have a roommate?

How often do you provide showers? Can I choose the time of day my loved one has a shower, or are showers provided only at certain times?

What toiletries should I provide?

Does the community provide incontinence products?

CHAPTER 23

Move-In Day

Keeping things positive

We've discussed the challenges that come with determining whether a care community is right for your loved one living with dementia. We have talked about ways to find a community that fits your family's needs. When it finally comes time to move that person, however, stress can hit you hard. You may second-guess yourself and all the progress you've made toward making this challenging decision—wondering if what you are doing is the right thing to do.

Madeline was furious. "Open the door!" she screamed, smashing her fists on the glass. "Open this door right now!"

Madeline's family had just moved her into our dementia care community. But her family did not make the move comfortable for Madeline. Instead, they had turned moving day into a complete disaster by telling Madeline that she had dementia and that she would be living in the community permanently. "Mom, you're here because you are sick, remember?" Madeline's daughter told her. "You have to stay here so that you'll be safe!" They upset her, and then they bolted for the exit.

These were not the right things to tell Madeline. Now she was angry, confused, and wanted to leave. Madeline did not believe she was sick—she felt fine! She did not want to be in a locked community where old and ill people lived. She was determined to get outside and get back to her house.

After giving her this information, Madeline's family attempted to leave the community without her. They *ran* for the door and closed it behind them before Madeline could catch up. "Hurry!" her daughter yelled to the rest of their family. "Let's go!" The older woman watched as they drove away and continued to beat on the glass with closed fists. It took hours to calm Madeline down and get her away from the door.

This was a tragic and avoidable scene that would have gone much differently had Madeline's family known how to handle the conversation. Although there is always a risk that a person living with dementia will be upset about moving into a community, especially at first, several tactics can help you get through this difficult day without turning it into a traumatic experience for everyone involved.

Remain Positive

Your "vibe" on move-in day, and on the days right before the move, has to be upbeat and positive. Even if your loved one isn't clear on what's happening or why, you can deeply affect the outcome based on how you handle it. If a family is positive and excited about the move, a person living with dementia will most likely feel the same. If a family approaches the move with caution, anxiety, and sadness, a person living with dementia will probably also feel distressed. So, it is imperative that care partners remain positive, even when the day becomes stressful. Remember, individuals living with dementia do not lose their ability to understand other peoples' emotions. If anything, they may become even more sensitive to them. To handle move-in day with grace, the family must first decide to be happy about the relocation themselves.

One of the worst move-ins I've ever witnessed was with Carl and his son, Trevor. Trevor was an anxious mess the day of the move. He came into our community with his dad by his side, both of them already arguing and tearful. My heart sank. I knew this was going to be awful. Despite our best attempts to calm Trevor's nerves, he continued to take out his anxiety on his already-upset father. "Dad! Relax, okay! Go sit down over there and stop talking to me while I fill out this paperwork!" Trevor yelled. We eventually separated the two of them—Trevor went with our marketing director to complete the paperwork, and Carl went to eat lunch with our other residents— but by the time Trevor and his kids had left, Carl was an emotional disaster. "Why am I here? Why did he leave me here?" Carl screamed, tears in his eyes, quickly pacing the hallway. I truly believe if Trevor had come in with a smile on his face—even if he didn't really feel that way inside—he could have "faked it till he made it" and created a much better vibe surrounding move-in day. His father fed off his negative energy—seeing that his son was upset, he couldn't help being upset about it, too.

Plan Ahead

There is nothing better than a good plan. A good plan doesn't mean that everything will go perfectly, but it does mean that move-in day has a better chance of unfolding peacefully. Madeline's family could have taken her to visit the community ahead of time to get her enthused about her new home. They could have shown her to her new room and presented it with a positive attitude. "Wow, Mom, this is a really nice room," they could have offered. "You have a beautiful view and plenty of space." They could have taken Madeline on a tour of the community, pointing out great spots to relax and enjoy activities and programs with other residents. They could have visited the dining area and tasted some of the food. By making the new environment an exciting and happy one, the family could have easily decreased Madeline's anxiety and anger. Even if Madeline was seeing the community for the first time on move-in day, she likely would have felt better about the move had the family approach it with positivity.

Some individuals living with dementia who are in the earlier stages may be willing and wanting to move to a dementia care community. Perhaps taking your loved one to a few communities to tour and empowering them to choose where they want to move can provide a more positive transition. Like most of us, people living with dementia feel good when feel they have some control over their own lives.

Another option, if your loved one is still angry or unconvinced about the move, is to consider blaming it on a third party. Telling Madeline that her "doctor thinks it's best she stay here" may have worked to allay her hesitation about the move. Pointing to a physical ailment, such as Madeline's recent knee replacement surgery, the family might have suggested to her that "the doctor wants you to stay here until your knees get better." Madeline may have felt better had she assumed that her move was not permanent and she could eventually go home.

When discussing options like these with your loved one living with dementia, remember that it is all about Embracing Their Reality. If you feel like it's important to tell them *your* truth about

the move, understand it may cause undue stress and pain. It can be devastating to find out that something is wrong with your brain and that your family is worried about your health care.

Telling Madeline that she would have to "stay there to be safe" and that she "lived there now" was also a mistake. By telling her these things, her family put a timeline on Madeline's stay, making the stay permanent. Madeline therefore became increasingly overwhelmed and confused. Many people living with dementia lose their ability to understand the passage of time. Two days can feel like an eternity, and two years can fly by. When asking those living with dementia how long they have lived in a community, do not expect an accurate answer. Many people will say things like "I have been here for three days" when they have actually lived there for six months. When Madeline learned the move was permanent, she panicked. That would be scary for anyone, but it is particularly terrifying for someone who does not understand the concept of time.

I suggest saying something like: "Mom, the doctor wants to observe you for a month or so while your leg heals." When we use a sentence like this, we are able to blame the move on a third party (the doctor), name an undefined amount of time (a month or so), and suggest that it is because of something physical that the person can feel or see (her leg). If she responds, "My leg is fine!" you can agree: "I know you feel better, but we all recognize how these doctors are—they love doing tests and observations!"

Madeline's family had a chance to help her look forward to living in the community, instead of turning it into a place where "sick people live." They could have presented it as a happy community where she would make many friends. They could have suggested that they chose it because she would enjoy herself there. Many people living with dementia in moderate to advanced stages lack the insight to realize there is anything wrong with them or others living with dementia. By telling Madeline she was sick, her family put her on the defensive. No one wants to believe they are sick or injured. After she heard that sick people lived there, Madeline became fearful and aggressive. She didn't feel as though she belonged in that environment and immediately began to fight back and attempt to leave.

Upon First Arrival

Another way to handle moving day would have been to provide Madeline with something to do once she arrived. Part of the move-in day plan should be discussed with the staff at the community. There should be a positive sense of welcome upon your arrival. Perhaps Madeline could have taken part in a meaningful activity, or her family could have introduced her to a new friend. While Madeline was happily engaged, they could have said goodbye for the day and left quietly.

The worst-case scenario is a family member or friend living with dementia that does not want to move—and understands that they are about to do so. If a person living with dementia knows that they are leaving a home behind, they may become upset and fearful. Although taking the above steps are important, sometimes a person just refuses to relocate, and they will not make the process any easier for their family. The best thing to do in this situation is to provide a distraction. Get the person with dementia inside the community, get them involved in a task or activity, and get the staff involved. Enjoy a meal together at the community or help your loved one begin a painting exercise. Once that person is engaged and active, it is time for the family to leave. Although it seems cruel, it is much better than telling a person living with dementia that they "live there now" or suggesting that they are there because of their dementia.

After a Move, When to Next Visit?

Some dementia community leaders will recommend that family members not visit a resident right after the move. Truly, though, there is no right or wrong choice of when a person should visit. Some family members visit right away, while others wait a week or two, to allow time for their loved one to adjust. This is an entirely personal decision. Some residents do better when they are given the space to get used to their new home. Others crave the comfort of seeing their families every day. In other words, it depends on how you and your loved one feel. Do your best, see what works, and adjust accordingly.

Managing Expectations

Like us, individuals living with dementia take varying amounts of time to adjust to life in a new place. Some people adapt immediately, whereas others can take days or even weeks. I once had a family member tell me, "Well, you've had my mom for three days, so I don't understand why she seems agitated when I visit." Three days is not enough time for most people to adjust to anything at all. Think about times you yourself have relocated. Did you immediately become comfortable with your surroundings when you moved to a new home or a started new job? With that said, most new residents living with dementia do not take more than two weeks to become settled.

If the first day at a dementia care community fails to go smoothly, families will often second-guess their decision. Some will say things like, "My mom isn't like the other people here" or "She isn't ready for this type of care." Typically, families overreact out of fear and guilt—they suddenly worry that their loved one is not ready for dementia community care. A catastrophic reaction by their loved one—screaming, crying, or arguing—can send many family members into panic mode. They imme-diately jump to the conclusion that every day will be like this and that they must move that person out.

Therefore it is so important to give a person living with dementia time to adjust to their new environment. The first day of any move will rarely go perfectly. Let the professionals at the community evaluate the new resident and watch their behavior over the first few days. Although you may be tempted to turn right around and move your loved one out of community care, it's best to wait at least a few weeks before making any rash decisions. Finally, once a person living with dementia is settled into a good community, their family should think twice before moving them again.

Putting It into Practice

Move-In Day Checklist

☐ *Toiletry items from home*: What did the community say you should bring? Do they provide towels and soap? What about toothpaste and toothbrushes?

Combs and hairbrushes? Make sure to pack those things.

- [ ] *Bedsheets and pillows*: What is available at the community, or what do you need to supply?
- [ ] *Beloved blankets or stuffed animals*: Bring a couple of favorite things, but be sure to have duplicates at home and label everything you bring in.
- [ ] *Furniture*: Most communities provide a bed, chair, nightstand, and maybe even another item or two. Know what the community is providing so that you don't end up with a lot of clutter and extra furniture.
- [ ] *Photos from home*: When bringing photos of friends and family, write the resident's name on the back. I cannot tell you how many times I've found photos of my residents' grandchildren floating around the hallways and been unsure of whose grandchildren they were.
- [ ] *Snacks*: If your loved one enjoys a certain kind of snack and it is okay with the community, send them in with plenty of snacks to share with their fellow residents. Nothing breaks the ice better than food.
- [ ] *A good attitude*: You don't have to be completely happy with a big transition like this, but if you can't pull it together for a few hours, send a friend or family member who can.

Managing Expectations

- *Addressing the move*: Any conversations you have with the person moving should include three things: blaming the move on a third party, suggesting that the timeline will be temporary but undefined, and then pointing to a physical ailment as the reason for the move.
- *Know who is assisting*: Who is going with you to make the move? Don't bring your entire family to help with the moving process, as this will cause unnecessary chaos.
- *Time the move*: I recommend moving someone around lunchtime, when they can immediately get involved with other residents and make new friends. A meal gives you time to finish setting up the room, and it gives them a chance to settle in.
- *Be cautious with valuables*: Don't send your loved one with anything irreplaceable, including wedding bands and rings. I recommend picking up a cheap replacement band and giving them that to wear instead of the real version.
- *Attitude*: Again, if you feel as though you cannot keep a smile on your face for the move, choose a proxy to go in your place. This is for your health and safety, along with the health and safety of your loved one who is living with dementia.
- *Check the room*: Visit the room ahead of time, so you know where you'll be setting up. Understand the space and size of the room, and take note of how much you can bring.
- *Don't panic if things don't go exactly as planned*: The unexpected is normal. Nothing will ever go exactly according to plan, but if you remain calm and focused, you will get through the day.

CHAPTER 24

Remember That Caregiving Is an Imperfect Science

Managing your expectations

Caring for people who are living with dementia is a challenging, imperfect science. I tell care partners that caregiving is more of an art form than it is a science. Once, while teaching a workshop I'd creatively named "Everything You Need to Know about Dementia," an older gentleman raised his hand halfway through my two-hour class. "Are you not going to talk about the neurology behind cognitive loss?" he asked, pen in hand. I shook my head and he looked genuinely baffled. "The title of this course is a bit misleading for advertising's sake," I smiled. "But, truly, even if I could tell you everything about the neurology behind a dementia disease, it wouldn't help you be a better caregiver. Dementia-positive caregiving is, at its core, an art form," I said. He seemed a little disappointed that we wouldn't be covering the detailed medical information behind dementia, but I could tell that he understood my answer. This is probably why when teaching groups I have found that students who come from a creative background tend to pick up challenging concepts quicker than those from a mathematical or logical background. I often joke with students at the beginning of my classes by asking, "Who in here is an engineer, lawyer, or mathematician?" Some students raise their hands, and I smile and laugh. "You're going to have a tough time," I say.

The Inner Workings of Care Communities

Caring for people is an imperfect science. You know this if you've raised or looked after a child. Looking after older adults living with dementia is even more imperfect. A common issue that I've encountered while working in senior living communities is that families expect perfection. Because the financial and emotional cost of moving a loved one is so high, they expect great returns—and I can't blame them! The residents of care communities have varying needs, backgrounds, and care plans. As I tell families, any good care community will do its best to take the weight off you, but sometimes it will fail to meet your expectations.

Now that I am not working in care communities full-time, I miss it. I loved being with residents all day: working hands-on with them, solving problems, and chatting with their family members. I often forget how stressful daily community care management can be. The residents were always my main focus, while residents' family members, my direct supervisor, and the regional management team vied for a close second place. I frequently had ideas and projects I wanted to implement but had to answer to not only my boss, but also to my boss's boss. Like any business, many facets go into making a care community run effectively.

Direct-Care Staff

At the best communities where I've worked, family members have close relationships with direct-care staff members. At some of the worst communities I've seen, families have little to no relationship with the care staff who look after their loved ones. Direct-care staff are the most important people at the care community. Without hands-on care staff, senior living couldn't exist. A huge problem in the United States—and probably other countries as well—is care staff turnover. Many care communities do not pay care staff what they are truly worth, and I personally believe that number should be much higher than most facilities are willing to pay.

The direct-care staff have the most challenging jobs: assisting residents with ADLs like grooming, bathing, dressing, toileting, and meals. They maintain relationships with family members and often become emotionally attached to their residents. When someone died or moved, it definitely affected me, but it did not affect me as deeply as it did many of my staff members. They were often devastated by continuous loss. Providing long-term, personal care to another person attaches you to them in a way that not much else can.

Social Workers and Memory Care Directors

I often have families ask, "Who do I talk to when I have dementia-specific questions?" I tell them to find the "me" at their loved one's senior living community, and by that I mean the person with the job that I always occupied. That will be the individual who runs the dementia-specific community or has a lot of involvement with both the residents and their family members. Sometimes this role is occupied by a social worker, but often it is someone with experience in dementia caregiving. They usually oversee the direct-care staff, activity staff, the activity calendar, and assist with move-ins and other big changes. I had different titles at different communities: dementia care director, memory care coordinator, memory support, among other titles. Effectively, they were all the same job description: to provide care, in any way necessary, to families and residents in the dementia care community.

Working in this specific role, I found myself wanting to speak to families about the idea of *imperfection*. The idea that, no matter how well you prepared, your day may not go exactly as planned. Although I did my best to make sure my staff stayed on schedule and we accomplished our tasks and goals for the day, something always happened—a fall, a new resident move-in we hadn't planned on, or perhaps a crucial staff member called out sick. It became clear to me that no matter how hard I worked to keep everything perfect, caring for human beings was distinctly imperfect.

The Executive Director or Administrator

The executive director or the administrator is the person who runs your loved one's community on a day-to-day basis. Some communities also have an associate or assistant director who serves as the main director's right hand. It is imperative that you meet—and like—the director at your family member's community. This person is responsible for the way the community is run, and they can affect the work ethic and attitudes around the facility. The best communities that I've worked with have excellent administrators, because the general feel of the community starts at the top and spreads from there. If your administrator is excellent, she will hire excellent management staff who will help hire excellent direct-care staff. If your administrator is less than amazing, the community is likely operate in a suboptimal way.

Typically, administrators and their staff answer to a regional team or a few regional members who do not normally work at the facility. The regional team oversees the larger community and may have multiple buildings in their region. The bigger the senior living company is, the more regional people will work there. This team manages everything from operational finances to big-picture dementia care. When it comes to making important decisions, such as whether to accept a potentially challenging resident into the community, regional teams can be very influential.

Other Positions

Every community will have similar positions, although the job titles may differ. Most places will have one or more nurses (depending on the size of the community), an activity director, a dietary director or lead chef, a few maintenance workers, housekeepers, a business office manager, one or two marketing directors, and potentially a few other administrative roles. All these positions work both independently and as a team to make sure the community runs as well as it can. For a business that runs twenty-four hours a day, seven days a week, communication between families and management becomes crucial. The best way to communicate with the management team is to find one or two managers who can assist you directly. Make those people the ones that you call or email every time.

Staffing Struggles

Staffing a care community twenty-four hours a day is demanding. Most care communities will have at least three shifts of workers throughout the day. Communication among the shift workers brings its own issues. Inevitably, communication errors and missed messages will happen occasionally regarding resident care. Because so many employees work in any given care community, a message has multiple chances to get lost. For example, a family member may ask a manager to ensure that third-shift workers clean his mother's room. Perhaps that manager didn't stay late enough to speak to the staff in person and forgot to write a note to third shift, or perhaps a staff member called in sick. Suddenly, the room does not get cleaned despite everyone's best intentions. A mixed or missed message is probably one of the biggest causes of confusion or mistakes in dementia care communities.

Care communities are notorious for high staff turnover rates. The hands-on caregivers in particular are typically underpaid. They resign often and are replaced as quickly as possible. Even at the managerial level, it seems as though people get traded between companies frequently. And even the best communities gain and lose staff members, which means rehiring and training are always going on. High turnover, in and of itself, causes some confusion throughout any care community.

Some, but not all, senior living communities will bring in what is often referred to as "agency staff" to help them with direct-care staff. This term really refers to staffing agencies, places that help senior living communities by filling in hands-on staffing needs when the community is short on staff. A senior living community can operate without the memory care director or the executive director for a couple days, but it cannot operate without enough hands-on care staff. Not only is it illegal, but it is also impossible to operate a facility without personal care for residents.

Imperfection Is Okay

Despite the things that can go wrong during your family member or friend's stay at a care community, the benefits of choosing community care far outweigh the negatives. As a caregiver, you will be free of the weight of having to provide for your parent, partner, adult child, or friend twenty-four hours a day. You know that, no matter what, your loved one is receiving care. They are with people who are at the same cognitive level and have similar needs. They have the ability to make friends and eat well-balanced meals every day.

For families looking to make a big move to a dementia care community, or for ones who have already made the jump, managing expectations is crucial. Sometimes, families will say things like, "He will live here for a little bit, and, when he gets better, he can move home." For a loved one living with dementia, this is probably impossible. Even with the absolute best care, he will continue to decline. Managing how we approach and understand senior living—recognizing that it is not a cure, but rather it is a safe place for someone to live out their life—is imperative before making a big move.

Putting It into Practice

What questions would you have for a dementia care director?

_____

What questions would you have for the executive director of a dementia care community?

_____

Perfectionism Homework

Make a list of what is essential for your loved one (such as help eating, toileting, etc.) and what is important but not essential.

_____

_____

_____

RESOURCES

Fazio, S., D. Pace, J. Flinner, and B. Kallmyer. 2018. The Fundamentals of Person-Centered Care for Individuals with Dementia. _Gerontologist_ 18, no. 58 (suppl. 1): S10–S19. doi:10.1093/geront/gnx122.

CHAPTER 25

Visiting and Saying Goodbye

How to visit and leave for the day without a battle

W̶e have a great time together, but when it's time for me to leave, I just don't know how to do it. It makes me want to stop coming in to visit at all," Wallace said with tears in his eyes. "I know that it's important I visit my wife here, but the act of leaving really takes a toll on my mental health."

Wallace is not alone in this sentiment. Visiting a person living with dementia—wherever that person may live—can be a challenge. I have heard many care partners express not only a fear of exiting for the day, but also a concern over what to talk about when they are there. From questions like "I do all of the talking—is that okay?" to "How do I walk out the door without starting a fight?" caregivers struggle with the acts of visiting and exiting.

How to Proceed

Before you walk in the door, create a plan for your visit, including how you'll finish the visit. A good plan goes a long way. At the end of the chapter I provide some tactics and strategies to help you and your family. Here are some important items to consider.

- Bring in something from home to talk about or do, such as a game or some tasks. I had a resident's family regularly bring their mismatched socks and laundry baskets to sit and fold with their loved one. It gave everyone a purpose and made conversation a lot easier.

- If you bring in a photo album, be sure to avoid correcting your loved one living with dementia when they mix up names or dates. Photo albums can be great conversation starters, but they can also be great argument creators.

- Talk about what you did that day. Although many care partners feel egotistical doing this, it's a great way to communicate with someone who doesn't (or can't) talk much.

- Choose a time of day that you will visit and a time of day that you will leave. Sometimes a half hour is a perfect amount of time for a visit. It doesn't have to be an all-day event.
- Engage your loved one living with dementia in an activity before you exit. As we discussed in chapter 23, meals are a great distraction that provide you with a chance to exit without a battle.
- It's best to visit earlier in the day. A late-day visit may mean you run into some sundowning behavior.
- Avoid using the word "home," particularly if you are their spouse. "I'm going home," usually signals to the other person that they are going with you.

A plan that you feel comfortable with can give you parameters to work within. For example, if you planned on visiting at 11:00 a.m. and leaving by 11:45 a.m., it's much easier to stick to the plan. Without creating a plan ahead of time, you may find yourself staying much longer, purely out of guilt.

Avoiding the Word "Home"

One of the hardest things about visiting a parent, partner, child, or friend in a dementia care community is saying goodbye for the day. Many visitors struggle with this. In an effort to tell the truth, family members will often tell their loved ones that they are going home after a visit. This typically begins a negative chain of events. For many people, especially romantic partners, "home" is a loaded word. When people living with dementia hear it, they typically think of the house they lived in with family members or a spouse—not their current care community. Although adult children can sometimes say they are going home without an issue, many spouses cannot exercise this same privilege.

If your family member or friend is not too advanced into dementia and is able to understand that you need to leave, then it's acceptable to announce that you are going home. Regardless, exercise caution when using this phrase, especially when your loved one first moves to a new community. It's important to test the waters and see how they react when you exit the community for the day.

"My mom keeps saying that she wants to go home," Eva complained. "She's been here for a month, and every time I see her, she asks to go home!"

Eva could not understand why, after all this time, her mother, Crystal, still asked about going home. What she didn't realize, however, was that Crystal never talked about home with anyone else. Seeing Eva reminded Crystal of home. Crystal's daughter was leaving for the day, so why couldn't they leave together?

Eva was so convinced that her mother hated the care community, she considered moving her out. It was not until she sat in another room and watched her mother eat dinner, happily chatting with other residents, that she realized her own presence probably caused Crystal's focus on returning home.

––––––––––––

When Eva wasn't there, Crystal never mentioned wanting to go home. But when her daughter showed up and mentioned "home," Crystal wanted to go, too.

When significant others living with dementia hear that their partner is leaving, they often head for the door, as well. Consider parties or events you attended together in the past. When you announced that it was "time to go home," you probably left the event together. This phrase still prompts a person living with dementia to believe that you are *both* leaving. It's understandable that your loved one living with dementia might get upset and angry when you tell her you are leaving but she cannot go with you.

Steps for Exiting without a Fight

First, unless this person is your spouse, try letting your family member or friend know that you are going home. As an adult child, you may find success in announcing that you are going home for the day. If this person is your spouse and they are confused about where they live, this method is not recommended. In any case, if this method doesn't work for you, drop it immediately. Understand that as your companion's dementia progresses, "home" may become a trigger word when it previously was not.

If telling your companion you are going home does not produce a positive result, tell them instead that you have to run some errands. Think of it this way: at some point in the future, you'll no doubt need to run errands. Saying that you have to go to the grocery store, visit the bank, or see another friend will eventually be true. So, say something like that as your reason for having to leave. By not saying that you are going home, there is less chance of hurt feelings. This method should work most of the time without any issues.

For some people living with dementia, that method will not work either. Your family member or friend may insist on going with you. They may say they enjoy running errands, and it would be nice to get out for a little while. In response, you could suggest you "do not have enough room in the car" or that you'll be back soon. Perhaps you have a meeting to go to, and it would not be appropriate for your loved one to come along. Maybe you are picking up a surprise (you can actually do that!) and you do not want them to know what it is. There are many ways to avoid telling someone you are going home for the day. The key is to remain creative and kind when finding a way to say goodbye.

For example, if your mom asks why she "has to stay here," you can give a number of positive responses. The doctor, nurse, or other staff members can help. Maybe she has a doctor's appointment today, and this is where it is. You could also suggest that this is where she will be eating breakfast, lunch, or dinner. If the next meal is coming up soon, this is a great time to exit the community. Maybe you can suggest to your mom that you are dropping her off at the community so she can lead an activity for the other residents. This works particularly well if your mom is used to being in charge of groups. Note that none of these statements needs to feel like a lie for either party.

Another easy way to say goodbye for the day is to get your family member or friend involved in an activity or event happening at the community. Maybe a volunteer is coming in to sing for the residents, or perhaps a few of the residents are arranging flowers. If your family member is happy and interested in a new activity, you shouldn't have difficulty leaving. You will feel better knowing that she is having a good time.

If all else fails, ask for help. Do not let your need to leave for the day cause a fight, and certainly do not avoid visiting because you dread the moment you have to leave. The staff at the community are there to support both you and the residents. Pick a staff member you trust, and let him or her know ahead of time when you will be leaving. The staff can help to keep your family member engaged or provide a hand to hold as you exit. No matter what, assure your parent, partner, child, or friend you'll be back to visit soon—and then follow through on that promise.

Putting It into Practice

List three things that you can bring with you on your visit that may make conversation a little easier.

_____

_____

_____

List three topics that you can talk about when you're with your loved one.

_____

_____

_____

Write down approximately what time you're going and what time you're planning on leaving.

In our dementia and improv comedy workshop, my friend Chris and I demonstrate a "good exit" and a "bad exit" upon visiting a loved one. Chris plays my dad, and we first demonstrate the "bad exit," which usually sounds something like this:

Me: It was great seeing you today, Dad! I have to go home now.
Chris: Yeah it was great. Sounds good, let me grab my coat.
Me: Dad! No! You live here now. You can't come with me. I just came to visit!
Chris: What do you mean? I want to go home, too. Let's go. I'm coming with you!
Me: Ugh, Dad, you have to stay here. I can't take you home with me.

The improvised fight usually continues on from there for another thirty seconds or so, as the audience squirms in discomfort. It's an uncomfortable scene to watch, because it's all too familiar for most people.

A "good exit" scene looks more like this:

Me: Hey Dad, it was great seeing you. I have to get going now.
Chris: Great, I'll come with you.
Me: I wish I could take you with me, Dad, but I have a doctor's appointment coming up and I don't want you to have to wait around with me in the waiting room. How about I come back and get you later?
Chris: Hmm . . . yeah, I suppose I don't want to wait around for the doctor with you. You'll come back for me after?
Me: Yes, I'll be back to see you later, Dad!

The "good scene" varies based on the answers we give each other, but they always revolve around the same concept: find a reason that Dad can't come home with me at that moment. This reason should make sense and apply directly to that individual; for example, something you know he won't want to do. Take note of something that may work for your exit strategy. Also, notice that in this scene's example, I did not say the trigger word, "home."

List three things your loved one would not feel like doing with you, such as going to the grocery store or waiting at a doctor's office.

List three things that may distract your loved one from wanting to leave, for example, having lunch at their community.

_____

_____

_____

RESOURCES

Mace, N. L., and P. V. Rabins. 2011. *The 36-Hour Day: A Family Guide to Caring for People Who Have Alzheimer Disease, Related Dementias, and Memory Loss*, 5th ed. Baltimore: Johns Hopkins University Press.

CHAPTER 26

Day Trips and Outings

Variety is the spice of life

O h, I just loved seeing those kids yesterday," Matilda exclaimed as we baked cookies with the other residents. Normally, Matilda's moderate Alzheimer disease prevented her from holding on to new memories. In this case, however, Matilda appeared able to recall an event that had brought her a lot of joy. Every Tuesday our group went to visit children at a local preschool. Even though Matilda could not recall what she had done every other hour of that day, she remembered visiting the children. It seemed as though the memory of the outing had found a special place to reside inside her brain.

The Importance of Outings

A s discussed in earlier chapters, when you are considering communities to join, it's imperative to look through their activity calendar. A place that lists the same four items on the calendar each day probably isn't a place that will offer stimulating outings for their residents—especially for their residents living with dementia. Communities that offer multiple monthly outings for residents living with dementia likely have a greater understanding and respect for their residents. It takes a proactive and dementia-friendly community to provide great outings for residents living with dementia. In other words, a community that offers multiple outings per month probably delivers better care overall.

These outings do not need to be long, and they do not need to be incredibly frequent. I have found that one outing a week is perfect. When I was in charge of making the community calendar, I looked for fun trips to take with my residents. Some of my favorites included:

- An outing for lunch
- A trip for ice cream cones
- A visit to the local animal shelter

- A trip to a to local preschool to read to children
- A bus ride through the rural parts of town

Early on in my career, I had the not-so-brilliant idea to take residents to the North Carolina Zoo, which was about twenty minutes from where our community was located. While the zoo was a great trip for families, it was a flop for the residents. There was a ton of walking, and as a result everyone was exhausted. We ended up pushing the residents in wheelchairs that the zoo provided, and my great idea for an outing quickly became a great example of what *not* to do.

Over time, I came to realize the key components to successful outings: they are short, suited to adults living with cognitive impairments, simple to organize, and do not include a lot of walking. For example, when we visited the local animal shelter, volunteers brought kittens and puppies to a quiet room. My residents were able to walk in, sit down, and have the animals placed onto their laps. The same trip can be a

success or failure depending on how it is organized. For example, taking a group of residents living with dementia on an unstructured trip to the museum may be challenging. Museums tend to involve a lot of walking, climbing stairs, and quiet reflection. People living with dementia may have trouble understanding the purpose of the trip or get tired from all the walking, which could make the experience stressful for those who aren't ready to return to the bus. But a well-organized trip to the museum that includes a tour led by a member of the museum staff who has been trained to work with people living with dementia should be fun and memorable for the residents.

"I'd like to take my dad out for the afternoon, but I'm concerned," Del said. "What if it's tough to get him back in the door when we're done with lunch? He does always ask about 'going home.'"

Positive dementia caregiving is all about trial and error. If you are unsure whether your best laid plans will work, go ahead and give them a try. If things don't go as planned, try again a different way, another day.

Holidays Outside the Community

Picking up a parent, partner, or friend living with dementia at his community and taking him to a holiday party can be a wonderful surprise. Remember that you will need to treat this trip like the other outings we've been talking about. People who have cognitive

impairments can easily become overwhelmed, so large parties may be challenging for them. Be sure to plan ahead. Ensure that your family member or friend has a quiet place they can go to get away from the noise of the party. It may also be useful to provide your family member or friend with a task. For example, if your aunt living with dementia can still set the table, ask her to do it. She will feel good about contributing and will probably fare better throughout the evening.

If your family always went to your aunt's house for Christmas Eve, sticking to that tradition might be a bad idea. If it seems like that particular tradition could be overwhelming for your loved one living with dementia, try something new. Above all else, recall that trial and error is your best bet for solving dementia-related challenges and concerns. It's not a bad idea to try the party at your aunt's house with a backup plan in mind, perhaps offering the back room as a quiet space for anyone who feels overwhelmed.

It is also important to talk to the rest of the family about how to address the individual living with dementia. Remind them that it's not appropriate to quiz your father living with dementia about his relationship to the rest of the family. Although he may recognize some family members, others may confuse him. Recall that Timeline Confusion may be at play here, and it's important to continue to live in his world and embrace his new reality. It is also best that the night end early for your family member living with dementia because sundowning may occur, especially if your loved one is overwhelmed.

For residents with mobility issues, trips outside the community pose additional challenges. Some communities may let you borrow a company vehicle, or they may provide a professional caregiver to drive you and your family member to and from the party.

The ability to remain active outside the walls of a dementia care community is incredibly important for people with cognitive impairments. Many residents look forward to outings with the community and those with family members. It's understandable that the first trip with a parent, partner, child, or friend may provoke anxiety for you and them. But following a few simple guidelines can help an outing go as smoothly as possible. People living with dementia deserve to live their lives in a fulfilling, engaging way that is not restricted to the inside of a building.

Putting It into Practice

Here are some tips and tricks when it comes to outings.

- If you are concerned about tackling a one-on-one outing with your loved one, try one with the senior living community. It gives you a chance to interact with your family member or friend outside the community without the stress of doing it alone.
- Plan ahead of time for the trip that you will be taking. You likely already know what types of trips your loved one would enjoy. For example, if your mom always loved going out for lunch, try that. Scope out a nearby restaurant ahead of time. Ensure there is enough seating and that the crowds will not be overwhelming at lunchtime. Make certain you can park close to the restaurant so you and your mom do not have to walk too far, particularly if she

has mobility issues. Once you both get inside the restaurant, be sure to sit close to a bathroom and an exit.

- Adapt the outing to suit your family member or friend's needs. At the restaurant, for example, a full menu of food options could prove overwhelming to your mom living with dementia. Instead of taking the menu away, modify the situation. Allow your mom to look at the menu for a few minutes. Then, offer her a choice of two or three items, and let her choose from that short list. Letting your mom look through the menu provides a sense of normalcy because that is the first thing most people do at restaurants. Still, you have successfully modified the trip by providing only a few meal options from which to choose.

- In restaurants especially, it is important to notify the waiter or waitress that your family member or friend has a cognitive impairment. There are a few ways to do this discreetly. You could pull the waiter aside and let them know that your mom is living with dementia. "My mom is living with dementia, but she is really excited to be here. I'm sure she would love to talk to you, but do not be alarmed if she seems a little confused," you could say. Recognize that some people are anxious about interacting with adults who have cognitive impairments, so it's important to phrase the dementia conversation with your waiter carefully. The Alzheimer's Association offers what it calls "Pardon My Companion" business cards. You can hand these cards out at restaurants or other public places you are visiting with your parent, partner, or friend. The card contains a brief explanation about dementia and may serve as a helpful

tool when you are out and about with your family member living with dementia. The cards are available online through the Alzheimer's Association.

- Don't take a person living with dementia to their old house, even for a brief visit. Once someone has adjusted to living in a dementia care community, a trip to their former home can be extremely confusing. They may wonder why they are visiting her old house, only to get back in the car and return to the dementia care community. For most dementia care community residents, this trip down memory lane will be greatly upsetting and confusing. In contrast, a trip to a relative's house may prove very pleasant.

- Keep the outing short and simple. The best outings I've orchestrated have been an hour or less, and there was always a distinct goal in mind. When we took a trip to get ice cream, we went in, sat down, I ordered everyone's ice cream, we ate, and we returned to the dementia care community. Everyone was thrilled with the trip, every time.

- Try to take outings earlier in the day. As the day wears on, many people living with dementia begin to sundown. The last thing you want is for your loved one or residents to start feeling agitated and irritable halfway through your excursion.

- Pack a car kit. The car kit should have extra medication, adult briefs if they use them, a change of clothes, snacks, and a couple bottles of water on hand. If worse comes to worse and your bus or car breaks down, a car kit will help ensure that we keep our friends living with dementia safe, comfortable, and calm.

- Recognize that you don't actually need to go anywhere to create a fun experience. If you are unable to take your dad on a real outing, try creating a trip inside the community. Call and ask the community's director if it is okay to eat with your dad in a quiet community spot. Pick up lunch or bring a homemade meal to enjoy with your dad in a secluded area. "Going out for lunch" doesn't mean that you need to go outside at all. For some people living with dementia, doing something different and enjoying a meal with you is enough.

RESOURCES

Alzheimer's Association. 2015. Seven Stages of Alzheimer's. www.alz.org/alzheimers _disease_stages_of_alzheimers.asp.

Alzheimer's Association. 2021. 50 Activities. https://www.alz.org/help-support /resources/kids-teens/50-activities.

Alzheimer's Association. 2021. Pardon My Companion Cards. https://www.alz.org /media/documents/alzheimers-dementia -companion-card-print-then-cut.pdf.

CHAPTER 27

Activities

Providing comfort and a sense of purpose

I have met many care partners, professional and family, who suggest that the person they are looking after "doesn't like to do anything besides watch TV or sleep." It's always frustrating for me to walk into someone's home, an adult day center, or a dementia care community and see adults living with dementia positioned in front of a television set. In chapter 11, on personal preferences, we focused on the idea that what makes a person an individual is their personality, the things they like and dislike, what they did and do for a living, among other quirks and routines. We can use this information to create individualized activities.

It's Not Just about Physical Care

Good medical care is extremely important in a care community, but it's not the only thing keeping residents from getting sick. Boredom and loneliness can be contributors to making someone ill. When I tour communities that boast wonderful physical care, I always look at their activity calendar. I want to see that there are multiple opportunities for engagement throughout the day, and that each day brings new activities and possibilities for the people who live there.

In my experience, the most important measure of any dementia care community is how it feels when you first walk through its doors. Trust your first impressions. Are residents engaged? Are they involved in activities or are they assembled in front of a television set? Is decade-appropriate music playing, or did the staff pick music they preferred? Or, worse, is the place silent? Are people smiling, laughing, and talking to one another—or are they asleep? How does the staff act when you come in the door? Do they greet you, or do they seem to ignore you? The answers to these questions can tell you a lot about what happens day to day in a community.

Initiating an Activity

I don't think he's getting enough stimulation where he's living now," Carol said of her husband. "This is a man who, even in retirement, found ways to stay incredibly active. He used to meet up with his friends at McDonald's every morning for coffee—even in the early stages of dementia!" she explained. "I'm concerned that I need to move him. I've talked to the activity director, but she doesn't seem to know what to do. Everyone just plays bingo all day, but he can't seem to follow along with the prompts."

Carol's story is all too common, unfortunately. There are plenty of wonderful dementia care communities that offer opportunities for engagement each and every day. But there are also communities that don't offer many activities, or at least not ones catered to people living with dementia. If the community isn't designed for people living with dementia, then it may not provide the emotional, social, medical, or physical care that individuals living with dementia require. In Carol's case, I recommended she look into moving her husband because he was in an assisted living building that didn't provide the necessary dementia care.

If moving someone to a different level of care is not an option, bring activities to your friend or family member's room directly. Although I've met care partners who hire outside assistance to do this, I feel that is not particularly cost-effective. Bear in mind that the amount and type of activity needed will vary depending on a person's type and level of dementia,

as well as what is an appropriate activity based on their personal preferences.

If you feel like the person you're talking to is going to say no to any activity you recommend, you simply need a new approach. Recall from chapter 11 that asking someone what they "like to do" usually doesn't provide us with much information. Along the same lines, we don't want to ask someone living with dementia if they "want to fold socks with us," as we will most likely hear something like "Why?" or "No way!" Instead, rephrase the sentence by asking for help. "*Can you help me* with this?" is much different than "*Do you want* to do this?" or "Do you *want* to help me?" When we ask someone if "they can help us," we make them feel necessary and important. The simple word change from "want" to "can" makes all the difference here. We are telling someone that we need them, not the other way around.

But if you don't get a response—such as the help you requested—try again in a different way. This time, initiate the activity yourself. If you're hoping the person you're working with will fold socks with you, try handing them a couple pairs to work on. Now, you're working alongside one another. Instead of asking, you're just engaging them in an activity. I often use this response when taking someone on an outing. "Come with me," I'll say, instead of asking if they "want to go," which usually just leads to questions about where, why, when, and how—all questions they quickly forget answers to.

Activity Ideas

There are many activities you can do alongside someone with dementia. Here are some that I have had a lot of success with. Many of these activities are portable and easy to initiate for both the care partner and the individual living with dementia. I recommend putting the items needed for these activities in bins (described in further detail at the end of this chapter) and bringing them on a visit or storing them at the community.

Sorting Socks

Generally, sorting socks is a fantastic activity for people living with dementia. Although laundry is typically not a favorite chore for most people, asking those living with dementia to help with sock sorting can provide them with a wonderful opportunity to be busy and engaged. Most people want to help others, and as the disease progresses, people living with dementia rarely get asked to assist with tasks any longer.

Folding Towels

Folding towels is the same type of activity as matching socks. People typically enjoy the activity because it feels useful and familiar—most people have folded towels previously in their lives. It feels like a necessary, important task to keep a household running. This type of activity can bring back memories of homemaking and raising children.

Matching Items

Some people enjoy strategy and thinking games, so matching cards or pictures is a good activity for adults living with dementia who can no longer complete more challenging brain games. An easy way to play is to lay colorful cards or pictures on a table and ask for help sorting through all of them. This can also work with holiday cards.

Matching Lids to Jars

Sorting through Tupperware may not be your idea of fun, but it gives people living with dementia the opportunity to be helpful and a welcome chance to do something useful. A mismatch of jars, containers, and lids can provide a person living with dementia a chance to sort and match the items. Note that glass jars may not be acceptable in all senior living communities, as some have rules or regulations against glass.

Building Blocks

More creative people, especially men who spent years building or working with their hands, may appreciate the opportunity to build or create things. It is important that the blocks or pieces used for building are not childish or too colorful. When given the chance to create something, it's amazing to see what people living with dementia can come up with.

Lacing and Tracing Kits

Sewing, especially threading a tiny needle, can present a huge challenge to a person with poor eyesight or arthritic hands. Lace and trace kits can be purchased online or in the game section of many stores. These kits usually include a few different shapes with holes around the perimeter. The user threads a colorful string in and out of these holes, moving around the shape. The motion is similar to sewing, but it is much easier to see and to hold.

Singing

Those living with dementia can often recall lyrics and melodies to favorite songs. It is amazing to see this in action. When it seems like other memories are gone, the ability to sing along to an old tune often remains. For many people in dementia care communities, the best part of any day is when an entertainer comes in to sing or play music. Pianists, singers, guitar players, accordion players, and dancers are sure to please at dementia care communities.

Fill in the Blank

Like music, fill-in-the-blank cards can work wonders for people living with dementia. For example, starting an old lyric like "I found my thrill . . ." gives someone time to fill in the rest of the sentence. "On Blueberry Hill!" he may say. Games that allow people living with dementia to think back to old sayings, phrases, and lyrics are usually successful and popular.

Completing Puzzles

Not everyone enjoys putting a puzzle together, but many people living with dementia relish the ability to complete something, especially when they have done it themselves. Puzzles for people living with dementia should have large, easy-to-see pieces and fewer than fifty parts that fit together. Anything bigger becomes overwhelming and can lead to frustration and anger.

Painting

A canvas and some paint give people who are living with dementia one of the most creative and entertaining things to do. "Paint whatever you like" is a great opener for this type of activity. It's interesting to see what a person will create when given the opportunity. If this activity becomes too difficult, something simpler, like painting the sides and roof of a premade wooden birdhouse, may work best. A few simple instructions are better than many complicated instructions. An invitation such as "Can you help me paint this?" receives a positive response from most adults with dementia.

Baby Dolls and Fake Pets

Much of a positive dementia care environment goes back to embracing the reality of the person living with dementia. A care partner who provides a baby doll to someone living with dementia is embracing that person's reality.

Many people living with dementia believe that baby dolls are real babies, and that stuffed animals are real animals. Care partners commonly ask, "Why does my loved one believe that a fake baby is real?" The answer lies in the way that dementia changes the brain. As the brain degrades, so does a person's ability to perceive, understand, and comprehend. Even if a baby doll does not cry, breathe, or require food or changing, a person living with dementia is unable to understand that the baby is not real. If it looks and feels real enough, it becomes real for them. As long as caregivers play along and treat the baby doll the same way they would treat a live baby, adults living with dementia may not be able to tell the difference.

"Hey, Seamus, can you watch this baby for me?" a staff member asked one of her residents. "I think she needs to go down for her nap soon."

Later that week, a staff member walked in to find Seamus cradling one of the baby dolls. He hushed the staffer. "Shh," he whispered, "I heard the baby crying."

Although these babies didn't actually cry, Seamus's brain created a meaningful moment for him surrounding the dolls. It made sense that the baby would cry—that is what babies do, after all. And because he thought that this baby needed his help, Seamus felt important and useful.

Providing dolls to a person living with dementia endows them with a sense of confidence and purpose. When asked to hold a baby, many people feel entrusted with a new responsibility, and people living with dementia are no different. It is still important for those with demen-tia to feel necessary and independent. Caring for a child, real or not, is a fantastic opportunity for a person living with dementia to be a caregiver again. Typically, baby dolls will also stir up memories. It's not uncommon to hear people reminisce about caring for their own children or what it was like growing up with their parents.

Stuffed animals—or real ones, for that matter—have a similar effect on people living with dementia that babies do. Stuffed animals are particularly useful for people in later stages of dementia because they neither require care nor do they accidentally scratch or bite the delicate skin of older adults. People who have grown up caring for animals usually love looking after a stuffed animal. Holding or cuddling a fake pet can bring immense comfort even to people who do not believe the animal is real.

"Oh," Gertrude whispered. "Is he for me?" She reached out to take the small stuffed dog. He looked remarkably realistic, even down to the softness of his fur.

"Sure, you can have him," I said, smiling as I handed her the stuffed animal.

Gertrude loved dogs. I knew she had owned a number of dogs in her life, and she was always excited when therapy dogs came in to visit with the residents. Recalling this, I hoped she would have the same reaction if handed a stuffed dog—and did she ever. Gertrude embraced the dog gently, holding him to her chest. "Oh, you are the sweetest thing," she whispered, closing her eyes and petting the dog's fur. "I will take the best care of you."

Some dementia care communities offer stuffed pets or baby dolls. For ones that do not, caregivers are welcome to provide a stuffed animal to their family member or friend. As long as these pets are labeled, they are unlikely to go missing, at least permanently. Some care communities also allow real pets to live with their owners, but in the later stages of dementia this becomes a problem. People living with cognitive impairments are often unable to get themselves to the bathroom, let alone care for a pet's waste. Sometimes, it is best to have a family member care for the owner's pet when the owner moves into a care community. Caregivers can then give their loved one a similarly sized stuffed animal, if they think it will comfort the person. In many cases, it does. If possible, the family can bring the real pet with them for a visit, as long as it doesn't cause distress or confusion for the person living with dementia.

Just as we introduce activities by asking, "Can you help me with this?" we want to introduce pets and babies in a similar way. "What do you think about this?" is a great way to find out where that individual's reality is. Asking this question prevents us from assuming that they believe the doll is real, or assuming that they think it's fake. When we ask what they think about it, we know right away if they believe it's real or not. If they think it's real, we go along with that reality. If they believe it's not real, we don't try to convince them otherwise.

Using What We Know about Personal Preferences

At one of my dementia care communities, the residents loved setting up for holiday events. One woman in particular spent about an hour meticulously decorating one of our Christmas trees. Clearly, she had done that in her own home and welcomed the chance to do it again. You may need to modify the activity slightly so the person living with dementia can feel successful. In this case, I handed items to my resident, and she put them on the tree. She was in charge of everything else, but because I handed her one ornament at a time, she was able to focus and avoid getting distracted or frustrated.

"When is payroll due?" James asked, walking into my office.

"What?" I asked, surprised by the question. I remembered, suddenly, that James had been an accountant his whole life. The well-dressed man was 100 years old, but he still believed that he had to go to work each and every day. "Uh, it's due today. Let me get you the paperwork," I offered. "Give me a few minutes."

James nodded and left. I threw together a spreadsheet with different numbers and printed it out. I hoped he would be able to add and subtract the numbers on the spreadsheet. I also found a pencil and a calculator and carried all of these to James. He took the materials and went toward his room. "I'm going to take these back to my office," he said, walking away.

About an hour later, James emerged from his "office." "I finished payroll," he said, smiling, as he offered me the worksheet and pencil.

––––––––––

James didn't want to fold socks or listen to music. He wanted to do what he had always done—he wanted to go to work. Working made James feel useful, smart, and successful. Allowing James to do something he felt was necessary and important was just as good—and perhaps even better—than any other activity he could have done.

Even though James didn't really do payroll, I still gave him a challenge. Although you may need to adapt your parent, partner, child, or friend's past career into something more manageable for them when they are living with dementia, they can still feel successful doing something they have always done.

Putting It into Practice

I highly recommend searching online for activities that meet the needs of older adults living with dementia. There are a number of excellent sources; here are a few of them.

Memorable Pets (memorablepets.com): stuffed animals and baby dolls that look real but do not move or make noise.

Relish (relish-life.com): activities for people living with dementia, each noted by stage of dementia and ease of use.

Mind-Start (mind-start.com): activities for adults living with dementia and my main source of fill-in-the-blank lyrics.

Joy for All Pets (joyforall.com): robotic stuffed animals that look real.

TomBot Robotic Animals (tombot.com): robotic stuffed animals that look real.

Pinterest (pinterest.com): search "dementia" and you'll find a massive collection of ideas for activities, but beware—these are not always designed by experts or even people who have tried what they're suggesting.

An Activity Box

Here is a way to create an appropriate activity box for someone living with dementia. You may be a direct-care worker, activity director, family member, or other relative of an adult living with dementia. You may be visiting with this box in hand, or you may be adding it to an activity closet where you can access it for many of your residents.

Step One: Find a box with a lid. This can be something you pick up from the dollar store, such as a plastic bin that comes with a lid. I find that items go missing at a much slower rate when they're secured in a storage container.

Step Two: Decide what type of activity box you want to make. I recommend that your first box be a sock-matching or towel-folding bin. I recommend baby socks, not only because they are cute, but also because residents are much less likely to try to put them on their feet.

Step Three: Pull apart the baby sock pairs and place them in the bin. We don't need a large amount of socks (ten pairs is a great start) because we don't want to overwhelm the person we are working with.

Step Four: Introduce the activity in a way that suggests you need their help, and not the other way around. "Can you help me match these socks?" you might ask. Put the bin in front of the person and dump the socks onto the table. If that seems like it will be overwhelming, sit down with the individual and hand them one sock at a time.

Step Five: When the matching is complete, celebrate the victory. Thank them for their assistance, and put the matched socks back in the bin. Be careful not to unpair them in front of the person who just took the time to match the socks!

Step Six: Unpair the socks in another area and place them back in the bin for later use. There's a good chance that a person with a severely impaired memory will be able to do the same activity again later that day.

RESOURCES

Green, C. R., and J. Beloff. 2020. *Through the Seasons: Activities for Memory-Challenged Adults and Their Caregivers*, 2nd ed. Baltimore: Johns Hopkins University Press.

Wonderlin, R., and G. M. Lotze. 2020. *Creative Engagement: A Handbook of Activities for People with Dementia*. Baltimore: Johns Hopkins University Press.

CHAPTER 28

Building a Dementia-Friendly Environment

What dementia-positive space looks like and how to create it

I remember a moment years ago when I was happily giving a tour of the dementia care community, where I worked, to a prospective family. I'd always enjoyed leading tours because I felt proud of what we had accomplished. I liked to show off our life-skills stations, which included the baby doll area, where residents would cuddle dolls; the desk and workspace for residents who felt as though they had to go to work; and the dresses, jewelry, and chest of drawers that looked like a woman's bedroom.

As I walked the family through our baby station, I pointed to the dolls. "Our residents really love this space," I explained, smiling. "They enjoy singing to the babies and rocking them back and forth in this rocking chair. Many take the babies back to their rooms. As you can see, we treat the babies as though they're real, because many of our residents believe that they are. Spending time with the babies can be incredibly calming for my residents, particularly for people with high anxiety." Turning to face the family, I saw the adult son shake his head.

"What a sad disease," he said angrily.

I was slightly stunned and didn't know how to respond. "But doesn't he see how wonderful this baby station is?" I thought to myself. It took me a moment to realize that many people who don't understand dementia could find this environment alien and bizarre.

We continued the tour, but my positive attitude was shaken. I was not sure what else to point out about the community, and I felt like I must have sounded naive, speaking so excitedly about baby dolls. At that point in my career, I had no easy way to explain to this man why baby dolls made my residents so happy. He probably thought we should have been trying to bring the residents back to our reality instead of embracing the world in which they lived.

Environment is an incredibly important part of positive dementia care. People living with dementia need—and deserve—to live in an environment that provides them with comfort, security, and happiness. That's why the best dementia care communities have spaces like the ones mentioned above. Life-skills stations, or places where residents can interact with relatable and comforting items, are integral parts of good care communities. When a person with dementia lives at home, it is equally important to create meaningful, pleasant spaces that are safe and affirming. These spaces make someone with dementia happy and eases their anxiety.

Immersive Worlds

When I think about what "positive dementia care" means to me, I picture an immersive environment designed specifically for people who may not recognize what year it is. This is a place where we are truly embracing the reality of the person or people living with dementia. The first—and probably the most talked-about immersive design community—is a place called Hogeweyk in the Netherlands. Hogeweyk is a senior living community designed specifically to meet the needs of older adults living with dementia. Their community is built to look like a town, where residents can access the grocery store, post office, movie theater, and more, all within the safe walls of Hogeweyk. The direct-care staff members who work there not only provide care to their residents, but also "work" in the stores, allowing their residents to continue living as they previously have. Another community, the Gateway Care Home based in the United Kingdom, boasts a train that serves tea to residents while they ride to their destination. The train doesn't actually move, but recorded images move past the windows as the sounds of a train chugging down railroad tracks play over speakers.

As the years go by, more and more places are recognizing a need for positive interior design in dementia care environments. I've noticed in recent years that the United States has started adopting this model of care, something that we were not focusing on when I started in my first senior living building full-time in 2013. Most dementia-specific communities in the United States are still built in the same way as assisted living and skilled nursing facilities: long hallways, apartment-style rooms, and random artwork. I recall a moment working in one community where I was told that interior designers were coming in to lay down new carpet and bring in new furniture. I was thrilled; we needed these items! Unfortunately, my hopes were dashed as soon as the designers came in the door. They brought carpet, furniture, lighting, and patterns that weren't designed with people living with dementia in mind. There is an art form to choosing dementia-specific designs, something we will cover in this chapter.

Lighting and Color

If you're choosing a care community for your loved one's care, you can't do much to change the entire building's lighting fixtures. What you can do, however, is keep an eye out for good and bad lighting. You can decide not to move someone to a community where lighting is poor. You can also bring lamps and better lighting to your relative or friend's room.

Changes in lighting strongly affect people living with dementia. Dark rooms with no windows are usually troublesome because they exacerbate a person's already impaired vision and depth perception. Our depth perception and balance change as we age, and they become perceptibly worse when we are living with a cognitive disability like dementia. In addition, a dark room implies that it is nighttime, making people tired and ready for bed. If you're wondering why the person you're caring for is lying in bed all day, look around at the lighting in the room. If it is dark in the room, would you be awake and ready for the day, or would you be lying down, too?

Color is important when choosing where someone living with dementia will spend most of their time. Even plate color affects how much we eat—even without a cognitive impairment! Blue is an appetite suppressant, and red is a color that's known to stimulate activity. Comforting colors are the goal when designing physical spaces for people living with dementia, so we wouldn't want to use red—an exciting color—all over the walls, but we would want to use it on plates to encourage eating.

A well-lit room with windows that is painted in warm colors does wonders for people living with dementia. This is important to keep in mind not only when visiting dementia care communities but also for people with dementia who are living at home. Lighting and room color affect everything from eating to sleeping. Our sleep/wake cycle is known as our circadian rhythm. Your circadian rhythm is a daily, natural process, which can be disrupted when dementia starts, making it harder to go to sleep and stay asleep, or even causing people to sleep for long periods. People in well-lit spaces are more likely to stay awake instead of nodding off throughout the day, which will help them to sleep better when it's time for bed.

Flooring and Patterns

Aylesa had younger-onset Alzheimer disease, a diagnosis she had received at the age of 58. Aylesa's children were grown and out of the house, and she lived with her dutiful husband and two cats. Upon a home safety visit, I inquired about the rug in their living room: an intricate, heavily patterned piece that stretched across the space. "Sometimes, when I walk into the room, the carpet feels like it's up to here on me," Aylesa explained, holding her hand up to her waist. "It looks like it's tall and three-dimensional . . . like I could walk into it or through it," she said. "But then I remember that what I'm seeing isn't real, and I force the thought to go away."

Because Aylesa was aware of her diagnosis, she was mostly able to speak about her experiences living with dementia. I knew that there would come a time, however, when Aylesa was no longer able to tell herself that the carpet wasn't in her way. I later suggested to her husband, in private, that he keep this in mind and remove the rug if it seemed like a distraction to his wife as her dementia progressed.

The perception of patterns and flooring can sometimes become distorted for adults living with dementia. Chairs, carpets, or tablecloths with patterns tend to confuse these individuals. For example, a carpet with a leaf pattern may encourage someone to bend down and attempt to pick up the leaves. A tablecloth with zigzag lines and bright colors may cause a person living with dementia to spend time playing with the cloth instead of focusing on a plate of food. Carpets with thick lines, or dark-colored rugs, can cause difficulties. Floor rugs, especially in dark colors, can cause increased confusion and may lead to falls. Some people living with dementia have difficulty discriminating between a hole in the floor and a dark-colored piece of fabric. Using fabrics and flooring devoid of patterns is important in dementia care environments. Shiny and reflective floors, like the ones that line hospital hallways, can also be a distraction, as they can appear wet to a person living with a cognitive impairment.

Music and Sound

Listening to music is an important part of many people's lives. For those living with dementia, hearing music can have an extremely positive effect on behavior. They often remember lyrics or tunes long after other memories have faded.

"I found my thrill on Blueberry Hill, on Blueberry Hill, where I found you," the residents sang in unison. Even if the lyrics had not been on the television screen, they would have known the song. To keep the positive energy flowing throughout the community, we installed CD players in most common areas. Pleasant, upbeat music played on repeat all day, every day.

Playing music in common areas for people living with dementia or even providing them with personal music players is a great way to keep them happy. Music has an impact on mood, and for people living with dementia, keeping the mood pleasant and comfortable is essential. In dining areas, communities can play music during meals, just as restaurants normally do. It's best if the music does not have lyrics because some residents will get caught up singing and forget to eat. Keeping the mood positive is an important step in getting residents to enjoy mealtimes and hopefully eat more.

Along these same lines, we don't want sound to be overwhelming. If you walk into a dementia care community and all you hear is yelling or loud noises, what do you think? It probably doesn't seem like a place that you want to move someone who is easily overwhelmed. Music not only calms and normalizes behavior, but it also drowns out other noises like food being served or toilets being flushed.

The Reward

Building a positive environment for a person living with dementia takes some creativity, but it doesn't necessarily require a lot of resources. For example, if you know that your mother living with dementia loves looking after children, she may enjoy a baby doll. Buying a realistic-looking baby doll and a couple of different outfits for it does not have to be expensive or time consuming. Even if your loved one lives in a care community without a baby station, there is no reason you can't suggest the community create a space for a crib. If that isn't possible, you could give your loved one a doll to carry with her and hold in her lap. Perhaps providing her with a CD or MP3 player would allow her to enjoy her favorite music. Choosing attractive pillows for your loved one's bed might encourage her to sleep there. There are many options for creating a welcoming environment where a person living with dementia can thrive.

Creating life-skills stations and modifying a person's environment can be enjoyable, especially when your efforts pay off. When you find that your mother enjoys her dolls, is less agitated, and generally seems happier, any time or money spent pays off tenfold. A person living with dementia requires a positive, engaging environment to live a happy, fulfilling life. People living with dementia may have a disease, but their lives don't have to end the minute they receive the diagnosis.

Putting It into Practice

Perhaps my favorite thing to do upon starting at a new dementia care community is to build life-skills stations. You can call them whatever you like; I think of these spaces as places that offer activities for residents. These activities are always available for someone to come upon. They can take up an entire room, a small part of a hallway, or even just a corner of a well-used space. If you're lucky enough to work in a dementia care community, you can help to build places like this. If you're a family member or friend of someone living with dementia and are looking to move them into a care community, keep an eye out for spaces like the ones below. Bear in mind that if the community doesn't have spaces like these, you can bring in fake pets, baby dolls, activity boxes, and more when you visit your loved one. Here are some of my favorite spaces to create.

- BABY DOLL NURSERY
  Items needed: baby dolls (two or three), crib or changing table, baby decor and signage, baby clothes and diapers, soft music
- PET SHOP
  Items needed: stuffed animals, carriers or pet beds, chew toys or cat scratchers, signage
- OFFICE SPACE
  Items needed: desk, notebooks, paper pens and pencils, computer or typewriter, calculator
- DRESSING ROOM OR LAUNDRY AREA
  Items needed: dresser or armoire, clothes, unplugged iron, ironing board, laundry basket, costume jewelry, scarves, hats, ties
- BUS STOP
  Items needed: bench, bus stop signage
- NURSING STATION
  Items needed: health care white coat, nursing cap, surgical masks, clipboard, stethoscope, pens and pencils, paper, blood pressure cuff

Choosing a Stuffed Animal or Baby Doll

How do you choose a life-like pet or baby doll that's appropriate? Let's look at a few guidelines.

1. Dolls designed for play by children are not appropriate for people living with dementia. We also don't want something that looks fake or silly. For example, I once went to a community where they said that they'd "tried baby dolls and it didn't work." I later found out they used Cabbage Patch dolls, which looked completely unreal. They also had a stuffed bear and claimed that was their attempt at "trying stuffed animals," when they would, in actuality, want a stuffed toy cat or dog.

2. Baby dolls should be about twenty inches in length and preferably have closed mouths. Babies with open mouths often get "fed" on a regular basis.

3. Generally, robotic pets are best for people in later stages of dementia. They are also more expensive and more difficult to clean in dementia care communities, where multiple residents will interact with them. Pets that do not move or make noise, such as those from Memorable Pets, fair well with people of all stages of dementia.

4. Consider your loved one's life history. What did the person like? Did they love raising children, or did they never want kids? Did they have a beloved dog growing up? Choose what you think they'd like.

5. Remember to ask the individual or individuals, "What do you think about this?" when introducing a stuffed animal or doll for the first time.

RESOURCES
Joy for All. 2021. www.joyforall.com.
Memorable Pets. 2021. www.memorablepets.com.
JC Toys Realistic Baby Dolls. 2021. https://www.amazon.com/stores/JCToys/page/0EDFCE80-127B-4795-808E-50149D7084ED?ref_=ast_bln.

PART V

Changes in Care

As a loved one's dementia progresses, care needs and attitudes change. In this section, I discuss the use of technology both for keeping someone safe and for enhancing their daily lives. I also discuss friendships, emotional and sexual relationships between people living with dementia, and when it may be time for hospice, among other important topics. The best plan is always to have a plan in the first place.

CHAPTER 29

When Technology Works and When It Doesn't

The role of tech in dementia care

I have split this chapter into two parts. The first discusses the benefits of technology, and the second discusses its drawbacks. I've done this because we can't talk about technology and dementia care without discussing the inherent problems in mixing the two. I have a saying that goes like this, "No amount of technology can replace human caregiving." This is an important concept for everyone who lives and works in dementia care to understand. I have often seen families of people living with dementia rely on technology to provide care for their loved ones. GPS tracking watches, cameras, medication reminders, tablets, fall alert devices, to name a few, all become heavily weighted crutches for desperate caregivers. "Mom is safe at home alone because she has a medical alert necklace," I've heard family members state. The problem is that these alert systems don't work if you take the necklace off or don't know how to press the button.

On the plus side, technology can augment human caregiving and bring joy to people living with dementia. The most popular example of positive technology in dementia care is a robotic seal named PARO that responds to touch and sound. In this chapter, we will review a number of positive dementia care programs and apps. When used appropriately, technology can improve the lives of caregivers and people living with dementia.

When Technology Is a Bad Idea

Because I work in dementia care and make that known online, I often hear from people in the tech industry. Once a month or so, I will receive a message that goes like this, "Hi, I've built an app that helps people with dementia. Can I send you more information so that you can review it for me?" When I first started in this business, I'd review every app that came my way. What I began to find, however, was that I ended up disappointing the developers of the apps.

I remember one in particular, from a man who had built a memory clock that worked with your tablet. It not only told you what time it was, but it also reminded you of any events that were coming up. In theory, this was a great idea: if your friend living with dementia couldn't remember the events coming up that day, here was a solution. There was nothing wrong with the application necessarily, but it certainly wasn't dementia-friendly. The person with dementia had to know how the tablet worked to find out what day and time it was! If you forget to charge the tablet, or if you forgot to look at it, the app was useless. And isn't that the whole trouble with dementia? People living with cognitive loss are not sure what they don't know. I told the man who sent me the tablet that I was sorry, but it just didn't make sense for people living with dementia. "This would be fine if it was used for someone in an early stage of dementia," I wrote to him. "Or, if it was used as a supplemental piece on top of actual caregiving. My concern is that a lot of families are going to see this and think that it solves the actual problem: that their loved one needs hands-on care."

Some families hear about medical alert systems and think they're the answer to all their concerns: with one of these devices, their loved one living with dementia can be safe at home alone. But this isn't true. I met a man who was taking care of his mother living with dementia in his family's mother-in-law suite. Jim's plan—to him, at least— seemed foolproof. "My mom wears a medical alert necklace, so she'll press it if she falls," he explained, pointing to his mother, now shuffling slowly out of her bedroom. "I don't think she will know to press it," I suggested hesitantly, biting my lip. "No, she will, watch this," Jim nodded to me. "Hey, mom," he called. "What's that necklace around your neck for?" His mom looked up, confused. "What necklace?" she asked. "You know, that one with the button," he explained. "What would you do if you fell? How would you get help?" His mother paused, unsure of how these two questions were connected, and thought. "I guess I'd call loudly for help!" She smiled, pleased with her answer. Jim wasn't satisfied, of course, and continued. "Would you press that button to call for help?" he asked, gesturing to her necklace. "Oh . . . yes?" his mom nodded. It was clear Jim's mother had no idea what the necklace was for, and certainly wouldn't be pressing it in an emergency to receive the required assistance.

I remember another time going to a client's house to see how he was doing. My client's daughter thought that she had it all figured out. She'd outfitted the whole house with cameras and put a GPS locator watch on her father's wrist. She'd labeled all the cabinets and put notes on the doors that read, "Dad, don't go outside." She meant well, but she was trying to solve an insurmountable problem like her father's dementia with the wrong kind of elbow grease. Her dad didn't need more technology or notes; he needed more caregiving. While the notes and the tech made her feel better, it didn't solve any problems. Her father never read the notes and often took off the GPS watch. When she was at work, she couldn't always check the cameras either, so it was easy for her father to wander outside without anyone stopping him.

There's a terrible, false sense of security that technology gives caregivers, especially family members of someone living with dementia. I think it's because a lot of programs or apps are advertised as a *solution* rather than an *adjunct* to care. I'm not suggesting you avoid using technology completely to help care for people living with dementia. What I am suggesting is that technology cannot be the only thing you utilize. While medical alert products, cameras, and GPS systems are excellent tools to enhance the way that we care for people living with dementia, they aren't the end-all-be-all answer to caregiving. They can't substitute for human-to-human contact. There might be technological breakthroughs in the future, like caregiving robots with artificial intelligence. For now, however, we have nothing that compares to the warmth and protection of human caregiving. There is no substitute for good, reliable, hands-on care in dementia caregiving.

When Technology Is a Good Idea

When we think about technology and dementia, we need to consider more examples than a medical alert necklace or a well-placed stair lift. What about the products that enhance the lives of people who have cognitive loss by engaging them in stimulating activities? We are seeing more and more simulations built into dementia-specific communities across the United States and in Europe. One community in the United Kingdom, the Gateway Care Home, has a train that residents can "ride" to new destinations. The train does not actually move, but houses and hills zoom by the window on a video loop, making it appear as though the train is headed through the country. Residents are greeted with train sounds, along with tea and treats they can eat during their ride.

Tablet or smartphone apps are also great ways to engage people living with dementia, so long as the applications are easy to use and understand. Look for apps that don't require a lot of instructions or buttons. Avoid traditional "brain-train" apps, which are designed for people who are not living with dementia. An app for someone living with dementia shouldn't claim to fix their dementia or even improve their cognition. Instead, the goal of a good dementia-appropriate app should be to engage them and enhance their life in a fun way. Below are some examples of tablet or smartphone-based apps that I recommend.

Dementia Australia's A Better Visit

A Better Visit is an app created for care partners to use with their loved ones living with dementia. It's meant to truly inspire a better visit when spending time together. The app has several easy games designed specifically for people living dementia, such as a coloring game, a maze, a fishing game, and more. It is peaceful, pleasant, and a lot of fun.

Virtual Aquarium

An aquarium, calming and colorful, without the mess! There are numerous virtual aquarium apps for your tablet or smartphone. No matter which program you choose, your loved one living with dementia can have an opportunity to care for fish without all the challenges that come with having an actual tank. This type of app is great for stress relief, especially for people who love fish.

Virtual Pets

When I was a kid, there were these great little toys called Tamagotchis. They were virtual keyring-sized games—far too small for my eyes, now, I'm sure—that allowed you to take care of a cat, dog, dinosaur, you name it. This technology is now outdated, and there are better, more vision-friendly options for your loved one living with dementia. Like the virtual aquarium, there are too many options to name them all. A few examples include Daily Kitten, where you care for a virtual cat, or Pet City, where you can choose from a number of pets.

Balloon-Popping Apps

A great task-oriented app is one where users can pop balloons or bubble wrap, or complete another repetitive motion. Balloon Popper is an app that allows you to do just that. It's easy to follow along and easy to set up. Like the other recommendations in the chapter, there are several other options out there to choose from when it comes to the right app for you.

Music and Breathing Apps

Personally, I like a nice breathing app. It sounds almost too simple, but it's not. We all know there's a positive correlation between emotional calm and guided breathing or meditation. These applications encourage you to breathe by visualizing the rate at which you inhale and exhale. Apps like these are perfect for combatting sundowning, particularly if you and the person living with dementia can practice breathing together.

Interactive Programs

It's Never 2 Late

My first 9-to-5 job in dementia care was at a Brookdale community in North Carolina. Not long after I started, we received a system called It's Never 2 Late. Brookdale had purchased the program and a few components that came with it. Never 2 Late connects through the community's television and other devices, such as a music-making machine or an under-the-desk bike pedal program. With the help of the person running the program, participants do a number of different activities already programmed into the system. We played music trivia, made Skype calls to residents' families, and created pages for each resident with their various likes and favorite programs.

PARO the Seal

If you haven't already, you must experience PARO the seal, invented by a Japanese company and sold all over the world. It is adorable but not cheap (it costs about $6,000). PARO comes in a few different coat colors and interacts with its user by making cute sounds and facial expressions. It responds to touch and sound, so petting PARO elicits a happy noise from the robotic animal. The company claims that PARO's users living with dementia are happier, calmer, livelier, and more interactive with others after using the robot.

Joy for All Pets

The Joy for All website advertises the slogan "No vet bills, just love." Much like PARO, these robotic cats or dogs respond to touch. Early in my career as a dementia care consultant, Joy for All sent me a cat to review. I have been bringing it with me to conferences and trainings ever since because it always gets a great response from the crowd. Many people who are not living with dementia have exclaimed, "Wow! I thought that was a real cat!" when they heard it meow from across the room.

Smartphone Apps

There are many apps built for caregivers to use alongside people who are living with dementia. A number of different organizations have reached out to me over the years to see if I'd review their apps. Often, the main goal of these organizations is to sell their product to home care franchises or senior living buildings. These applications usually work on tablets and offer the user the ability to track and record information about clients or residents. Users are able to record information like a residents' likes, dislikes, history, and more. Some can save someone's favorite music artists or clips from their favorite movies. A good example is RemindMe Care, an application developed in the United Kingdom.

There is no shortage of great technological advances that we can use to enhance the lives of people living with dementia. There are also a number of options to make caregiving easier, especially in home care settings. Knowing all of this, it's imperative that we use technology with the goal of enhancing caregiving. There is still no substitute for human interaction in dementia care.

When you get a chance, look through your smartphone or tablet's app store or browse the Internet for various tech related to dementia caregiving. You'll be impressed and probably surprised by how much is out there.

CHAPTER 30

When It's Time for a Dietary Change

As dementia progresses, many people need dietary changes

Eating and drinking are necessary parts of our lives and can even be hobbies for some people. Many adults take pleasure in trying new types of food, cooking, and baking. Unfortunately, dementia can affect the way someone enjoys and experiences food. A person's ability to taste certain things, chew certain foods, or swallow becomes affected as dementia progresses. Typically, in the later stages of dementia, a person will struggle to ingest most food. Families need to be prepared to handle the dietary changes that come with a person's cognitive loss.

When a person living with dementia moves into a care community, a nurse, doctor, or speech therapist will assess their diet and ability to consume food and liquids. This professional may recommend that a person living with dementia follow a diet different from what they are currently eating. For some residents, this may include food items that are easy to pick up, such as sandwiches or other finger foods. Some residents may be on a diet of only pureed foods. Residents who are in advanced stages of dementia typically have difficulty swallowing and feeding themselves. They may require a diet that helps prevent choking during mealtimes. Some families find these changes difficult to accept. But realize that altering diets allows residents to safely get the right amount of nutrition.

Mechanical Soft or "Ground" Diet

Jessica sat at the table, trying to eat a sandwich that her daughter had brought. The sandwich looked delicious, but Jessica seemed to be struggling: the thick bread and the meat inside proved difficult for her to chew. Jessica took small bites, chewing hard, but took the bites continuously until there was a significant portion of food pocketed in her mouth. Still, Jessica's daughter insisted that she knew her mother's needs. "Mom never eats enough," Julie said. "That's why she's losing so much weight! Look at how rail-thin she is."

Jessica was too thin, but Julie misunderstood an important issue regarding her mother's eating: that she could not physically eat—at least independently—some of the things that were put in front of her. Still, Julie protested that Jessica was choosing to eat too little. "That's why she's here," Julie said, holding up her hands for emphasis. "She needs the staff to push food and liquids in her."

Julie did not understand that her mother had lost weight partly because she could not easily eat certain foods. The family was doing what they thought was right—putting plenty of food in front of her—but it was the wrong type of food. Jessica actually needed to be on a mechanical soft diet, which consists of foods that are soft and easy to chew. This type of diet can include hard-to-chew foods like steak, but the steak needs to be finely ground before it's served to the individual on the dietary restriction. Because Jessica was living with dementia, she couldn't express that she was having trouble eating. She also may not have understood why she was not able to eat the food her family gave her.

Puree or Liquid Diet

Kara had always loved chocolate, which her son remembered. As Kara's dementia progressed, however, she could no longer feed herself or eat the same foods. She was at a significant risk for choking, so her diet had been changed to pureed food. Kara's son lived in another country, though, and while we'd communicated that her needs had changed, Kara's son did not realize the extent to which this was true.

Kara's birthday was approaching, and her son sent her a box of chocolates in the mail. "Happy Birthday, Mom!" the card read. I sat and stared at the box of chocolates: I knew that she could not enjoy them, at least not in this form. The chocolate pieces were going to be sticky and hard to chew, which meant they'd be impossible for Kara to eat safely. Still,

the last thing that I wanted was for Kara to miss out on her favorite food, especially since they were a birthday gift from her son. Suddenly realizing there was another option, I contacted our chef. "Can you puree these chocolates into liquid chocolate for me?" I asked.

"Sure," she said. "I'll add some whipped cream so it's not just pure chocolate. Bring me the box and I'll get that together for you." Our chef pureed the box of chocolates with some whipped cream and a little bit of milk. I took the candied mix up to Kara, and with some help from the staff, she was able to enjoy her birthday gift.

Kara was fortunate because our kitchen staff was able to puree her box of chocolates. This may not be an option in every facility. Be sure to review your family member or friend's diet with her care providers to determine what types of gifts or treats are appropriate. This will ensure she's able to enjoy your gift safely. It is important for families to respect residents' diets in dementia care communities. Although you may like the idea of giving your dad cheese cubes to snack on, they may be too chewy for him to handle. Realize that an accidental dietary mishap can be fatal to a person who has trouble swallowing.

Pureed food may not look appetizing, but today there are more attractive puree diet options. There are now puree molds and premade pureed foods. You can obtain a pureed chicken breast that is in the shape of a chicken breast, instead of slushy off-white chicken puree in a bowl. Note that individuals living with later stages of dementia may not be turned off by the look or feel of food. But people living with earlier stages of dementia who are at risk of choking may not want to eat something that doesn't look tasty. For them, these pureed foods that look like solid food might be the answer.

Finger Food Diet

Ted was always up and about. It was difficult for him to sit down and enjoy a meal with his tablemates because he was so distractible and physically active. He was also not able to feed himself using utensils. Ted could often be seen picking up a fork, looking at it, and putting it down again. Sometimes he would place his utensils next to other people's plates, probably thinking that they must belong to someone else, as he did not know what they were used for. Still, Ted was not at the point where he wanted or needed a staff member to assist him with eating: he could still pick up food with his fingers.

Knowing this, the doctor recommended a finger food diet for Ted. When the community had chicken breast, the staff gave it to Ted on a bun. When the community had soup, they put it in a mug for him to drink. Ted got to enjoy the same foods as his fellow residents, and he was able to do so in his own way. Eating utensils had become a real challenge for Ted, since he didn't know what they were or how to use them. Although eating on his modified diet was not as clean and tidy as using a knife and fork, Ted was able to eat independently. Ted's diet also allowed him to get up and move around, taking the food with him. His nutrition wasn't at risk because he was able to get the right amount of food in the right way for him.

Modifications to Utensils and Dishes

Many people, especially in the later stages of dementia, will lose their ability to eat "cleanly." They may make messes on the table and all over their plates. Some people may be on soft-food diets and also misunderstand how to use a fork or spoon. Still, they want to eat independently and choose to continue eating using their fingers and hands. In situations like these, a plate guard is a good option. A *plate guard* is an object that curves around a plate and prevents food from falling off the edge of the plate. While this may look odd to you, recognize that it is an important way for a person living with dementia to remain independent. With a plate guard, there is no need to assist them. Instead, they are in control of what and when to eat.

In some instances, helping a person living with dementia take a few bites of food may then cue then to continue eating. For example, some people living with dementia will be able to eat with a fork once a care partner helps them put food on the fork. If your dad has trouble using a fork, you may choose to put your hand under his hand and guide the fork to his mouth. After a few tries, your dad may be able to do the motion on his own. For many people living with dementia, the skill of eating by oneself is not completely lost until very late in the disease process. Some people, though, need a little bit of help to get started with eating a meal.

Some great adaptive utensils and dietary products have made it to the market in recent years. For example, there are "no-spill" cups that don't tip over, made with people who have Parkinson disease in mind. There are also plates that are made to stick the table. For someone with tremors or trouble controlling their movements, these modified dishes are perfect. Additionally, there are foam pieces that slip right over utensil handles. These enlarge the handles on forks, spoons, and knives, making them easier to control in arthritic or shaky hands. More ideas to make eating less frustrating are presented at the end of the chapter.

Importance of Snacks and Water

Urinary tract infections are incredibly common among residents in senior living communities. One of the reasons for this recurring problem is residents don't drink enough water every day, causing dehydration. Most people living with dementia will not remember to drink water, and some people will not remember that they need to eat. This is why it's incredibly important to encourage liquids and food on a regular basis. Instead of asking, "Do you want something to drink?" I recommend just filling a glass of water and handing it to the person you are looking after, as there is a good chance they would refuse your offer, not even recognizing they are indeed thirsty. I have also met people who "don't like water," and in these circumstances, I recommend serving 100% juice or juice with a low sugar content.

One of my favorite activities in dementia care communities was snack time. I would push the snack cart around, handing each resident a snack that fit their dietary profile. Most of the residents would never have asked for a snack and were thrilled to receive one. It wasn't that they weren't hungry; rather, they did not remember to think about food. I found that regular snacks between meals decreased agitation, especially in the late afternoons. An after-dinner snack could be crucial in preventing sundowning.

Not Eating

People living with dementia will eventually lose the ability to eat independently. No amount of cueing or reminding can help a person who has forgotten how to take food in. In situations like these, it is imperative that a caregiver assist that person with the entire meal. In dementia care communities, professional caregivers know who needs assistance with eating. They help residents with eating and drinking throughout mealtime. Care partners are encouraged to help residents living with dementia feel empowered while eating. For example, the person living with dementia can hold on to a caregiver's hand or wrist while the caregiver holds the utensil. This allows the person to feel as though they are still involved in the eating process—it is not happening *to* them but *with* them.

Some people living with dementia will refuse to eat or will begin eating only certain foods. When this happens, find a solution by becoming a dementia detective (something we talked about in chapter 12). Many people living with dementia will begin craving sweets at some point in the disease process. Although this seems odd, it occurs because, as dementia progresses, a person loses the ability to distinguish between tastes. Sweet foods may become more palatable to people living with dementia, even if they didn't indulge in sweets earlier in life.

There are several ways to encourage a family member or friend with a cognitive impairment to eat more. Ensure that they are eating in a well-lit environment. Limit certain distractions in the area, such as overly stimulating music or excess numbers of people. We offer more ideas at the end of this chapter. Recognize that when it comes to eating and dementia, people's needs change as the disease progresses, so they may approach food differently. Not only do they have to eat food in different forms in order to eat safely, but also their desire to eat at all may go down.

Recognize that the end-of-life process always includes the slowing of food intake. People who are in the first stages of the dying process will begin to refuse food, pushing plates or bowls away. This is normal. We should not force someone who is dying to eat or drink when it seems as though it is making them more uncomfortable.

Putting It into Practice

Here are some tips to encourage eating:

1. *Make sure that what you're offering is sweet and tastes good.* Many people living with dementia eventually lose their ability to taste foods that aren't sweet. Also, did your loved one like that food or drink before they got dementia? Don't introduce new items, like extra protein, into the diet. Instead, focus on what they enjoy.
2. *If your loved one is forgetting how to use utensils, instead of fighting it, adapt.* Switch to a mug for drinking soup if using a spoon and bowl is too difficult. Offer food they can pick up with their hands—a burger and fries is finger food!
3. *Offer small meals throughout the day instead of big meals two or three times*

a day. Snacking is easier because a person can get enough water and food without sitting down for a whole meal.
4. *Don't ask if they are hungry.* Instead, just present the food and beverage. "Here, this is for you."
5. *Offer more water throughout the day.* One thing caregivers sometimes forget to offer is water. Don't ask, "Are you thirsty?" but instead hand the person living with dementia a glass of water without asking.
6. *If your loved one is having trouble swallowing, consult a professional to help adjust the diet.* You may need a mechanical soft (ground) diet or a puree option. You may also need to add thickened liquids.
7. *Eat together.* People living with dementia have an easier time following cues when they can mimic others.
8. *Change the color of the cup and plate.* Make sure that the cup and plate are a different color than the actual meal— red is a great option. Blue actually discourages food intake.
9. *Turn on some music (without lyrics).* We're often used to eating meals in restaurants or at home with some music on in the background. Play music without lyrics, though, since singing may distract from eating.
10. *Make some modifications to plates and mugs.* Below is a list of some adaptive dietary equipment.
11. *Serve one part of the meal at a time.* Think about this as the way you'd eat in a restaurant: you would have an appetizer, then the main course, and then desert. It can be confusing to a person living with dementia if they get a whole tray of food at once to move through.

Adaptive Equipment

Spill-proof cups and mugs: cups and mugs that do not tip or do not spill if they tip.

Divided plates: plates with sections for each food, particularly useful for pureed foods.

Plate guards: guards that hook on to plates to keep food on the plate and reduce mess.

Nonslip mats: mats that make it more difficult to knock plates or cups off the table.

Plates with lip: plates with built-in plate guard.

Foam handles for utensils: foam that covers the utensil's handle to make it easier to hold.

Weighted utensils: heavier utensils that are easier to grasp.

Bendable utensils: utensils that can be bent to fit a person's hand.

Elastic cuff for utensil: cuffs that clip to the utensil and then to the individual's wrist.

RESOURCES

Memorial Sloan Kettering Cancer Center. 2021. Eating Guide for Pureed and Mechanical Soft Diets. https://www.mskcc.org/cancer-care/patient-education/pureed-and-mechanical-soft-diets. This website provides an excellent overview of pureed and mechanically soft foods, including recipes. Although it is written for individuals who have cancer, the material is applicable to those with dietary changes seen in dementia.

Stelter, J. R., and R. Wonderlin. 2021. *The Busy Caregiver's Guide to Advanced Alzheimer Disease*. Baltimore: Johns Hopkins University Press.

CHAPTER 31

Friendships and Disagreements among Residents

Bonding through friendship is imperative for people living with dementia

When families ask me, "Why should I move my loved one into a dementia care community?" I always put social interaction at the top of my list. People living in dementia care communities benefit by being around others at their cognitive level. This gives many residents a chance to make friends, create relationships, and have meaningful interactions each day.

I have to imagine that if you're living in a place where everyone is more cognitively alert than you are, your daily interactions could feel overwhelming. This is one of the main reasons that residents with dementia from a community without dementia-specific care eventually move into a dementia-specific care community. They no longer fit in with the rest of the population. They aren't able to make many of their own decisions and care for themselves, which makes social interactions more challenging. As I mentioned in another chapter, some cognitively able individuals will bully or belittle adults living with dementia. In contrast, when adults living with dementia live together, they tend to accept each other more easily. They don't notice each other's memory impairments and speech challenges the same way cognitively able individuals do.

The roommates were inseparable. If one was sleeping, the other was sleeping. If one was on her way to the dining room, the other was right beside her. Vera and Molly were the best of friends. Vera was not as advanced in her Alzheimer disease as Molly, but the two knew each other—there was no doubt about that. Vera knew Molly's name, while Molly did not actually seem to know Vera's. Molly often referred to Vera only as "my roommate," but that distinction worked well for the pair.

"Hey! That seat is saved for my roommate!" Molly often called out to a resident who had taken Vera's seat on their couch. Granted, the couch didn't actually belong to them, but if the pair sat anywhere, they sat on the same two-seater sofa.

"Oh, don't worry, Molly, I'll just sit over here," Vera would offer.

"No, no, this is your seat, and this knucklehead is sitting in it!" Molly would hiss, pointing at the resident who had adopted Vera's seat. Molly was deeply annoyed by someone co-opting her friend's spot. It was always difficult for me to hold back a small laugh when I watched this interaction take place.

Whenever we took the residents for an outing, Vera ensured that Molly was beside her. "Where's Molly?" she would ask. "She likes ice cream outings, too. I had better go get her!" Vera would go back to the couch to get Molly. The pair would ride on the first two seats of the bus, and Vera would always help Molly up the stairs of the vehicle.

Molly needed Vera for reminders and assistance. Vera leaned on Molly mostly for friendship, because Molly was unable to provide many cues or reminders owing to her advancing Alzheimer disease. The two widowed women had loving family members, but their families had lives of their own and could not visit too often. In lieu of family, they had each other.

One day, Vera's family decided to move her to a new community. They were relocating and wanted to move her, too. "We aren't worried," the family said. "Vera will eventually forget who her friends are at this community, anyway." I feared what would happen to Molly once Vera moved. Molly relied on Vera's cues and directions to get through the day. She needed her best friend beside her.

The day Vera moved, something changed in Molly. She no longer fought for that couch seat. Often, Molly did not even sit on the couch they used to share. Instead, she migrated from seat to seat, almost aimlessly. Although she could not explain what was missing, something was clearly wrong. Something had changed.

"We'll tell her that Vera is on vacation," my staff agreed, planning ahead in case Molly asked about her friend. It would have been heartbreaking to tell Molly the truth of our reality.

Molly became focused on physical things, like the missing furniture in her bedroom that she once shared with Vera. "What happened to the furniture in here?" she asked. And then, concerned, she turned to me. "Is someone going to sleep in here with me tonight?" Tears welled up in my eyes as I realized that she did not want to be alone.

———————

Molly never asked about Vera, probably because she could not quite place the loss. We found her a new roommate, someone who could also provide cues and direction, but it was not the same. Although the new roommate was kind, the pair did not connect on the same level that Molly and Vera had.

While Molly could not quite place Vera when she was no longer physically present, it did not mean that Molly would not recognize Vera immediately whenever she saw her. Even in a large crowd of residents, Molly could find and point out her friend. Molly didn't know Vera's name, but she knew that Vera was her friend and her roommate. The ability to recognize a person is preserved long into the progression of Alzheimer disease. Because people living with dementia are at a high risk for depression, making connections with others who are living with dementia is invaluable. Humans still desire friendship and love, even in the midst of cognitive loss.

———————

Disagreements with Other Residents

Living in close quarters with other people inevitably brings about its own challenges and tribulations. Like everyone, those living with dementia have certain people they prefer over others. Unlike everyone else, however, they face an added struggle: cognitive loss. This may cause residents to snap at each other, argue, and occasionally start physical confrontations when they never would have done so before dementia.

"Give me back my blanket! That is my blanket, and you stole it from me!" Arlene cried out, trying to snatch her handwoven blanket back from Marla's grasp.

"No it's not!" Marla yelled. "My momma made this blanket for me, and if you try and take it I'll slap you right across the face!"

Marla was not just threatening Arlene with words. Marla was the type of woman who meant what she said, and the staff knew she would slap Arlene without hesitation. I quickly intervened and assessed the situation. I knew the blanket did belong to Arlene, and Marla had a tendency to enter other residents' rooms and take their belongings.

She went into other people's rooms so often that many of the residents began to remember her. "Hey! That's the lady who takes my stuff! Get her out of here!" some of the residents would yell when they saw her approach.

In order to get the blanket back without confrontation, I calmly asked Marla to join me outside. The temperature was over 90° Fahrenheit in the courtyard, and I knew Marla wouldn't care about that blanket for too long in that kind of heat. We talked for a couple of minutes outside. "Hey, Marla, do you want that blanket?" I asked. "It's pretty warm out here!"

"No, it's too hot for this thing." Marla shook her head, handing me the blanket.

I eventually returned the blanket to Arlene. But it was just a small victory in the ongoing battle of dealing with Marla's behavior. Eventually, after a number of documented incidents like this, we were forced to move Marla out of the community. Her verbal threats of violence—and sometimes physical attacks on others—were not a match for this community.

Marla's case is an extreme example. Our staff could not keep her or the other residents safe, especially when she angered them so often. All the residents' family members knew her, and many of them feared what she'd do next. Marla was an incredibly confrontational person, so it was tough to have her around so many other people.

When a resident constantly gets into trouble with others, alternative placement may be in order. Typically, it takes multiple complaints or a serious incident before a resident is asked to leave. Because it's so hard for families to find dementia community placement, many communities hesitate to force anyone to leave. If the reasons are serious enough, a community can relocate a resident even if the family is against it.

In many cases, disputes between residents arise because one or both of them has a medical issue that hasn't been solved. For example, urinary tract infections (UTIs) cause behavioral changes in many residents. UTIs affect people living with dementia differently than they do people with normal cognitive functioning. In people living with dementia, UTIs commonly cause increased confusion, agitation, anxiety, anger, and sudden mood swings. The good news is that most UTIs clear up quickly with medication, and typically any issues between residents dissipate.

Handling Aggression in Others

If an issue between residents occurs while you are visiting, try not to get involved. Something you say or do could anger another resident further, and you may find yourself a target. For example, if you are visiting your father in his dementia care community and you see another resident, Mrs. Blackwell, is not her usual pleasant self, let a staff member know. If she and your father have always gotten along well but she now seems aggressive and upset, this could signal something seriously wrong with Mrs. Blackwell's health. Sometimes families notice behavioral changes before staff members, especially if their loved one has close friends in the community. And if another resident acts aggressively toward you or your family member living with dementia, seek help immediately. Do not attempt to calm the person down or prevent a verbal fight. Remember that de-escalation techniques are different in dementia caregiving, since we cannot use logic to try to convince someone they should calm down.

Recurring Problems

If an issue between your parent, partner, child, or friend living with dementia and another resident seems ongoing, talk to the executive director or whoever runs the community. It is not fair for your loved one to live in a community—and for you to pay for it—where there is continuous conflict. Ongoing issues are rare, although they most often occur between roommates who don't get along. Usually, one of the roommates desires more space than the other. For example, if Milton feels very protective over his room, he may not understand why his roommate Matthew is always there. Milton believes the room belongs only to him, so he picks verbal fights when Matthew enters the room. Ongoing squabbles like these do not happen often, mostly because of the nature of dementia: many residents lack the ability to remember small quarrels that they have with others, but they may recall if another resident upsets them on a regular basis.

Bridget was terrified of Louis. In a previous argument, he had threatened to hit her. Although Bridget's short-term memory was poor, she could recall a strong emotion such as fear. Bridget still harbored bad feelings for Louis, even if Louis did not feel the same. In fact, Louis seemed to have forgotten the confrontation completely. Still, Bridget refused to enter a room where he was sitting unless she had a staff member by her side. This became an issue because Louis liked to sit in common areas.

Instead of getting involved in the dispute, Bridget's daughter did the right thing: she talked to the staff. They were able to assure her that Louis had not made any threats for quite some time but that they would continue to look out for her mother's health and safety. Bridget's daughter also made sure to greet Louis with kindness and let her mother see this. Louis always responded positively, and Bridget's fear of the man began to dissipate. As the months went by, Bridget's fear subsided. Eventually, she was able to enter rooms where Louis sat without an issue.

———

Bridget's daughter dealt with the problem by employing two important techniques: (1) talking to staff members and (2) showing kindness and courtesy to Louis. Bridget saw these positive interactions, and they helped her get over the issue.

Although many people living with dementia get along wonderfully, the chance always exists that two people will not connect. If an issue develops between your family member or friend living with dementia and another person, remember to take the high road. Instead of intervening and potentially making the problem worse, look to the staff to help ease your concerns. Recognize that two people who are living with dementia—even if they are the same age and gender and share similar backgrounds—are not going to have the same experience with cognitive loss. Remembering this can make your interactions with other people who are living with dementia a lot easier.

Putting It into Practice

Be sure to document any aggression that you notice between residents.

What happened?

Between whom?

_____

On what date and at what time?

_____

Who else was present?

_____

How was it resolved?

_____

RESOURCES

Pearce, B. W. 2007. *Senior Living Communities: Operations Management and Marketing for Assisted Living, Congregate, and Continuing Care Retirement Communities*, 2nd ed. Baltimore: Johns Hopkins University Press.

CHAPTER 32

Sex and Sexual Orientation

The birds and the bees at 83

Although many people feel uncomfortable talking about emotional and physical relationships between older adults, the reality is that love and sex do not suddenly stop at a certain age. Nor do these things cease because a person is diagnosed with dementia; they just become more challenging when dementia enters the picture. In this chapter, I'll be discussing sexual relationships between people living with cognitive impairments, sexual relationships between a person living without dementia and a person living with cognitive impairment, changing relationships, and lesbian, gay, bisexual, transgender, queer, questioning, intersex, asexual, plus (LGBTQIA+) conversations in dementia caregiving.

Having dementia does not mean that a person loses the desire or ability to maintain a romantic relationship. For many people living with dementia, romantic companionship is still incredibly important. Numerous types of romantic relationships can begin between residents at senior living communities. While some are physical in nature, others are not. Care partners can significantly improve their parents, siblings, or friends' lives by accepting their romantic relationships with others.

Sex and Dementia

In dementia care, sexual relationships between consenting adults can be a challenging topic. It is also not a topic many people want to address head-on. "My partner isn't able to engage with me like they used to," one caregiver told me, shyly, after a workshop. "I want to talk to our doctor about it, but I feel awkward."

When one person is living with dementia, the line between sexual *consent* and sexual *assault* can blur. People living with dementia, especially later in the disease process, may not have the ability to consent to sexual activity. As a result, couples need to reevaluate their physical relationship because of dementia's impact.

An individual used to having a regular sexual routine can find this challenging. Saying something like, "Well, they used to always _____" is not a good way to decide about a person's new sexual wants and needs. What they used to want and need has changed and is now potentially impaired because of cognitive loss.

Ken and Mary Lou had been married for fifty years. Their relationship had always been happy and loving, and so had their sex life. As they aged, both began to have cognitive loss, but Mary Lou's impairments were significantly worse than her husband's. Though they moved into the same room in the same community, Ken did not need the same level of care that his wife did.

Mary Lou was confused. At times, she was not quite sure who her husband was. He seemed to be much older than she believed she was, so she had trouble placing him on her timeline. Ken, however, always knew who Mary Lou was and wished to have the same relationship with her that he had always had. The problem was that Mary Lou no longer had the ability to consent to sexual activity. She could not really say yes or no because of the way dementia had impaired her brain.

Even when it was clear that she could place him, and knew that he was her husband, the line felt blurry for the staff. "I can't tell if she wants to have sex with him or not," one care staff member noted. A few times the staff had to separate the couple, because they felt, at that moment, that sexual contact was inappropriate for Mary Lou. Because Mary Lou was no longer sure how to engage in sexual activity, her husband was occasionally pushing her into sex without her consent. Although it was awkward, the staff did their best to keep an eye on the couple's physical encounters.

The issue of sexual consent is an important and confusing part of dementia care. It is not a black-and-white issue, and there is no one-size-fits-all answer. Although Ken and Mary Lou had a fulfilling sex life in the past, Mary Lou's new brain state prevented her from enjoying or understanding what was occurring. It became an issue, then, of timing. At times, Mary Lou could consent to and enjoy sexual activity with her husband. At other times, Mary Lou was not capable of consent. Like Mary Lou, some people living with dementia do not necessarily have the ability to understand what is going on before, during, or after sex. So how does one know if their loved one can consent? At the end of the chapter, we provide more information on how to help decide if someone is able to consent to sexual activity.

Changing Relationships

For some partnerships, intercourse quickly becomes a non-option. This may be because of one person's cognitive impairments, or it may be solely due to their physical inability to have sex. Whatever the case, it's important to find ways to engage with a partner romantically, even if they cannot engage with you sexually. This may mean that you start engaging in more comforting touch, such as holding hands or linking arms. Even a reassuring touch can turn someone's bad day around. The desire for human contact is far from lost among people with dementia, even if sexual activity is out the window.

It is not uncommon for the partner without a cognitive impairment to lose their desire to have sex with the individual living with dementia. There may be a case where the person living with dementia wants to have sex, but the person without dementia is no longer feeling the same desire or attraction to their partner that they used to feel. This situation is perfectly natural. Becoming a care partner takes significantly more investment and weight than being someone's romantic partner. For some people, this changed role may make sex feel awkward or unenjoyable with the person who is impaired.

"I feel like I'm caring for my dad all over again," Deirdre sighed as she talked about her partner. "I still love him, but I don't feel the same sexual or physical attraction to him anymore. It makes me feel terribly guilty."

Deirdre's story is not unusual. I recommend that anyone who is feeling guilt—of any kind regarding caregiving—be sure to seek help. Walking around with the constant burden of guilt is not healthy, and it will not help you be the best care partner you can be. Deirdre eventually found a therapist with whom she met twice a week. She later reported that she was feeling better about her changed relationship and was also beginning to accept her changed feelings for her partner.

Inappropriate Sexual Comments or Activity

It's possible that the individual living with dementia exhibits sexually inappropriate behavior or speech. This is not uncommon in dementia, particularly for people living with frontotemporal dementia (FTD). This type of sexual behavior may manifest itself in awkward comments to wait staff at a local restaurant, unwanted advances toward staff members at a dementia care community, or unwanted sexual advances with a romantic partner. No matter what the actual behavior is, understand that the individual who is doing it is unaware that their behavior is inappropriate and unwanted. This means that saying "Ew! Go away!" is not an appropriate response to an unwanted advance. Instead, calmly tell them that you do not want to be on the receiving end of that kind of behavior. "Please stop doing that. You're making me uncomfortable" is an appropriate response. Remember that this person has a brain disease and should be treated with respect and kindness despite their actions.

For some individuals with extreme hypersexuality, a trip to the doctor is warranted. For example, if your loved one is constantly trying to push others into sexual activity, particularly if these other people are individuals who cannot consent, speak to the physician about options, including possible medications, to calm their libido. Again, the person making these advances is most likely unaware that their behavior is not desirable. Yelling at them or physically pushing them away—unless, of course, you are being physically attacked—is not appropriate.

New Love in Senior Living

One of the biggest challenges that care partners encounter is seeing their married family member or partner begin a relationship with another resident. Under normal circumstances, a married adult having a relationship with a person other than her spouse is considered adultery. Dementia is not a normal circumstance, however. As always, it is imperative to embrace the reality of the person living with dementia. Some people living with dementia are unable to remember that they are married, while others believe that another resident is in fact their real spouse.

> Gloria and Joe were inseparable. The pair did well together because they shared the same level of cognitive functioning. The only problem, however, was Joe was still married. Joe's wife, Sue, visited the community often. She knew about Joe's relationship with Gloria, but there wasn't much she could do. Even though Joe enjoyed his wife's visits, he always went back to Gloria's side after Sue left the community for the day.
>
> In Joe's mind, Gloria was his wife. He saw Gloria every day, her room was next to his, and they sat at the same dining room table. Joe also knew who Sue was when she came to visit. Joe seemed to believe that Sue and Gloria were the same person, and in his world, that made sense. Both Gloria and Sue had blonde hair and a similar body type. When Sue was not there, Joe's brain made sense of her absence in his new home by making Gloria his wife. Although it confused outside parties, in Joe and Gloria's world, their relationship made perfect sense.
>
> Joe would introduce Gloria as his wife to staff members. "Where's my wife?" he would ask, and the staff would point to Gloria. If Sue was there, the staff members would point to Sue. Because of Joe's memory impairment, he was unable to make this connection. To him, both women were his wife, and both women brought him happiness.
>
> Sue was surprisingly tolerant and even accepting of her husband's relationship with Gloria. She understood that his brain forced him to live in a different world than hers. In some ways, Sue was even thankful for Gloria—Gloria kept Joe company when she could not be present. Although Sue

found it hard at times, she knew Joe loved her more than anything. In fact, he loved her so much that his brain created a copy of her when she could not be there.

Not everyone is as accepting of a loved one's new relationship as Sue was with Joe. Sue's ability to turn her husband's relationship into a positive event made their lives less dramatic. Instead of being upset and jealous, she understood that her husband was living with dementia. Sue knew that Joe was confused about his relationship with her because she was not always by his side. Sue decided to be happy and accepting, rather than angry, that this confusion had occurred.

New Partnerships in Senior Living

In some cases, people living in dementia care communities will partner up. These partnerships may be fleeting, as some residents will constantly forget who their new partner is. Other partnerships will remain in place for long periods. In these situations, it's up to families to support their family member's decision to be in a relationship. This is a frustrating and embarrassing topic for many people to discuss, particularly if you're caring for your parent. Recognize that the staff at the community expect these kinds of relationships to begin and do not judge you or your parent for allowing them to continue.

Michelle had never seemed to notice Russell before. They had both lived at the community for years, but recently the staff noticed that the two were a couple. Before she noticed Russell, Michelle mostly kept to herself. She was a kind and incredibly well-dressed woman of 81 years, but she never wanted to join in community activities or outings. "Oh, no, honey, I think I'll just stay behind here," Michelle would say when asked about going out for lunch or ice cream.

As soon as she began dating Russell, everything changed. The pair could be found strolling the hallways together, hand in hand. They did everything together, including going on outings. Russell had never been much for trips outside the community either, but together the pair was up for any and all adventures. It was clear to everyone they brought out the best in each other.

Michelle's daughters were more than happy about her new relationship. "Mom is doing so well now! We love that she's become close with Russell," they explained. The same could not be said for Russell's daughter, however. She was obviously distraught over her father's relationship with a woman who was not her mother. Even though Russell's wife had passed away years before, Russell's daughter didn't think her father should have any more romantic partners.

Eventually, Russell's daughter decided to move him to a new community. Although she claimed it was because the new community was closer to her home, it likely had something to do with Russell's relationship. Immediately after Russell moved out, Michelle's attitude changed. "He'll be back, I know it," she would say. Even though she was living with dementia, Michelle spent quite a long time mourning the loss of her boyfriend.

———————

Michelle and Russell made a fantastic pair; unfortunately, Russell's daughter didn't see it that way. She was bothered, like many family caregivers, by her father carrying on a romantic relationship in a senior living community. What she could not understand was that her dad still needed love, companionship, and affection. Even though Russell was living with dementia, he was still an adult capable of making his own decisions regarding companionship. Russell had chosen another cognitively impaired adult with whom he could have a consensual relationship. Moving to a new community likely affected his mental state. He was probably more confused and lonely than before. Dementia and depression often go hand in hand, and encouraging positive relationships between residents can be a great way to combat emotional decline.

Although it is your prerogative to try and prevent your loved one's relationships with others, it is best to accept that you cannot truly stop them from engaging with other residents. You are not there all day, every day, and your family member or friend living with dementia is going to do what they want to do. Remind yourself that your family member is an adult and that it is not your job to manage their relationships with other adults—even though they are cognitively impaired.

Evolving Identity

Interestingly, some people in dementia care communities who once identified as heterosexual may end up identifying otherwise. This is not because being around the same sex changes a person over time. It's also not because a woman living around many other women realizes that dating a female may be numerically easier. If someone begins identifying as a part of the LGBTQIA+ community, it is most likely because they have felt this way throughout their life. Now, living with dementia, their "filter" is gone, and they become more of who they always were. Their previously felt need or desire to hide their true feelings is no longer present. It's doubtful that anyone living with dementia would come out and say, "I'm gay now" but instead may begin acting more openly on their feelings and emotions. Now, in dementia care, they are comfortable to be their true selves.

This scenario could be jarring for a family or care partner who always believed their loved one was heterosexual. "I did not see that coming," Will laughed kindly, motioning to his father, holding hands with another man at his table. Will was taking it in stride, but he admitted that it made him uncomfortable at first. "I just kept thinking about how mom would feel," he said. "And then I realized, it's okay. She isn't with us anymore, and dad still deserves to be happy and to be his true self." The fact that Will was able to accept his father's lifestyle was instrumental in keeping his father safe, happy, and secure in his dementia care community. This also cemented the strong bond the two of them continued to share.

Ellen had always been attracted to women but had never told anyone. She had grown up in the 1940s, a time when people could not safely share their LGBTQIA+ orientation. She did what society expected of her: she married a man, had children, and lived out her life. Now that Ellen was living with Alzheimer disease, the part of her brain that told her to hide her sexual attraction was gone.

The staff was slightly confused when Ellen began holding hands with another female resident in the community. They were more surprised when they spotted the pair kissing in the hallway. "I thought Ellen was married to a man!" one staff member commented.

———

SAGE Advocacy and Services for LGBT Elders is a national organization that promotes healthy aging and conversations about sexuality. They have tools and information for families and older adults to learn more about identifying as part of the LGBTQIA+ community in later life.

Be aware, too, that someone who no longer feels the barriers to being open about their sexuality may also lose the same barriers to expressing their gender. For example, I worked with one community who had a male resident who began dressing as a female. He had never previously done that, so his family was confused. As it turned out, this man had always felt that he was female but never felt as though he could express it. Now, unconfined by his brain's filter, he was able to be fully true to himself.

Respect

Although a relationship between older adults is an issue that many families do not enjoy discussing, it is important to have this discussion. Because the people in senior communities are adults, they are able to decide with whom they will or will not have a physical relationship. Staff will notify families immediately following a sexual encounter between their family member and another person.

Family caregivers then bear the difficult task of deciding to encourage or dissuade this relationship between their family member and the other person. One of the best ways to decide what to do is to talk to the staff at the dementia care community. If a relationship is positive, full of joy and consent, caregivers may find that respecting their loved one's desire to engage in that relationship is the best thing to do. Even if that relationship is uncomfortable to think about or discuss, emotional and physical relationships between residents can be influential, powerful, and loving.

Putting It into Practice

"Can my loved one consent to sexual activity with me or another person?"

1. Are they in an earlier stage of dementia? (Moderate or beyond stages mean that they no longer recognize that they are impaired and cannot live independently and safely. At this stage they will need much help with daily activities.)

_____

2. Do they recognize their sexual partner most of the time?

_____

3. Are they able to verbalize "yes" and/or initiate sexual activity with positive physical affirmations?

_____

4. Do they seem interested in sexual activity?

_____

If you answered yes to the above questions, your loved one can probably consent to sexual activity without an issue. If you answered no to some but not all of these questions, this does not necessarily mean they cannot consent, but it does mean you should evaluate what you wrote and why. As I often tell families regarding sex, as long as we are taking into account the individual's best interest, we are using positive dementia caregiving techniques. If the answer is no to all the above questions, this person cannot consent to sexual activity.

"How do we separate two people who are engaging in sexual activity but shouldn't?"

- Decide if these two people are able to consent to sexual activity. If the answer is yes but they are in an inappropriate space (such as the common area of their dementia care community), quietly escort them to private space.

- Decide why you feel as though their sexual contact is inappropriate. Is it because you yourself are uncomfortable seeing it, or is because one or both parties cannot consent to sexual activity?
- If you still need to break up the activity, do not yell, act disgusted, or call attention to the people engaging in a physical act. Instead, calmly redirect one or both of them. A great example would be to say, "Sarah, can you come with me? I have something I need your help with." A best practice is to pretend as though you are not bothered by, nor even notice, that they were engaging in a sexual act. We do not want them to feel embarrassed or uncomfortable.

RESOURCES

SAGE Advocacy and Services for LGBT Elders. 2020. LGBTQ Aging: The Case for Inclusive Long-Term Care Communities. https://www .sageusa.org/resource-posts/lgbtq-aging -the-case-for-inclusive-long-term-care -communities/.

Yee-Melichar, D., C. Flores, and A. Renwanz Boyle. 2020. *Assisted Living Administration and Management: Effective Practices and Model Programs in Elder Care*, 2nd ed. New York: Springer.

CHAPTER 33

When It's Time for Hospice

End-of-life decisions are hard to talk about

"I think that we should talk about getting your mom onto hospice services," I said, doing my best to broach the subject with care. "What?" Ed replied, surprised. "My dad was on hospice, and I knew when he needed it—I don't think my mom is there, just yet," he said. "Your dad had COPD [chronic obstructive pulmonary disorder] and heart failure," I explained. "The end of person's life with dementia often looks a lot different than how we expect it to appear."

After some convincing, Ed took my advice, and we looked into hospice care for his mom. Sure enough, a hospice physician declared her ready for hospice services. Although he'd been hesitant at first, Ed was thrilled with the care his mom began receiving—and all for zero financial cost to him. A couple days after his mom started hospice, Ed asked the provider team about an oxygen machine to help his mother breathe easier. In no time at all, the machine arrived at her community, again, free of charge. The hospice team provided adult briefs, gloves, and cleansing wipes for the caregivers to use, which were all items he'd been purchasing himself in bulk.

Hospice sent an aide to the dementia care community twice a week to check on his mom and assist with showers. As she began to decline further and enter the active dying phase, hospice came more often, helping at the bedside to keep her clean and comfortable. Finally, as she passed away, a hospice nurse came to pronounce death. "I'm so glad that you told me about hospice when you did," Ed said.

———

What Is Hospice?

When most people hear the word "hospice," they cringe with fear. Traditionally, hospice has been for people within six months of death. In reality, however, individuals can stay on hospice for much longer and even sometimes *improve* under hospice's care—known as graduating from hospice—because hospice provides them with the extra assistance they'd been needing. Hospice is a holistic, team-based approach for individuals with a life-limiting illness. "Life-limiting" means that the illness is terminal, and a physician or team of providers believes the person is declining and has approximately six months or less of life to live. A hospice team is an on-call service that is made up of physicians, nurses, social workers, direct-care aides, volunteers, and spiritual counselors. The team works to provide patients and families with pain control, symptom management (such as assistance with nausea or anxiety), and personal care, such as bathing and feeding.

Some people believe that one has to physically move to a hospice building to receive their services, but this is far from the truth. Although some hospice organizations have a physical place patients can move to, most hospices come right to the patient. Dementia care communities, and assisted living or personal care communities for that matter, frequently use hospice compa-nies that will come to the patient. It is not uncommon to see a couple of differ-ent hospice organizations working in the same care community, as families are able to choose a hospice care organ-ization that appeals to them. Usually, hospice companies will provide showers to their patients even though the care aides at the community can help with resident showers. Many hospice compa-nies will cover the cost of adult briefs and other incontinence supplies as well as wound care products. Some hospice organizations go to care communities to provide education to the staff about their services, and they will often host a bingo game, provide snacks, or even bring in pets for pet therapy while there.

When someone is undergoing hospice care, they cannot seek treatment or solutions for illnesses. For example, a person on hospice cannot also be receiving chemotherapy or radiation for cancer, but they can continue taking medication for pain related to the cancer. Hospice companies do not want their patients visiting the hospital without speaking to their hospice physician first. While this may seem odd, it makes sense. If you are visiting the hospital, it is probably because you want to fix something about your illness. Hospice is for individuals who are no longer seeking treatment or solutions to an illness, but rather are looking for comfort and symptom management.

Be aware that should an emergency—such as a fall or stroke—happen while someone is in hospice care, the hospice company must be notified immediately. You can no longer take the individual to the hospital for treatment. Instead, you or the person's dementia care commu-nity would call their hospice. Hospice will decide whether the individual needs to go to the hospital. Families who choose to send their loved one to the hospital, regardless of what hospice thinks, will have to revoke hospice for them to receive treatment in hospital. Revoking hospice requires a family to complete paperwork to get their loved one back onto hospice care after they have been released from the hospital.

Hospice is paid for by Medicare, Medicaid, the Veterans Health Adminis-tration, and most private insurers. In other words, hospice is free for the person and person's family who is receiving the care. I have heard many families remark that it seems almost "too good to be true," but it is true. It does not matter what someone's income or status in the community is when it comes to receiving hospice care. If an individual is not on Medicare or Medicaid, there are still options available to them, such as submitting information to the hospice organization regarding a financial hardship in the hopes of receiving full or partial financial coverage.

What Is Palliative Care?

Palliative care and hospice are not the same thing. Although most hospice companies provide palliative care, others do not. Also, palliative care is not just for people who have a life-limiting illness the way that hospice is. Instead, palliative care can provide relief from physical pain and mental stress. The goal of palliative care is to manage symptoms of an illness or injury; relieve pain and discomfort; improve quality of life; and meet the emotional, social, and spiritual needs of the patient. While both hospice care and palliative care provide comfort, palliative care can begin at diagnosis and occur in conjunction with treatment, while hospice care begins when treatment has stopped. For example, a person with a recurring wound may seek help through palliative care. The person with the wound doesn't have a life-limiting illness, but they do have a lot of pain and a wound that needs treatment, including regular dressing changes from a trained professional. Put another way, a person who wishes to receive palliative care doesn't need a doctor to certify that they have a life expectancy of six months or less.

When Should Someone Consider Hospice?

Ed had trouble identifying when his mother was entering the later stages of her disease process. Because he did not see her every day, he often missed the small changes that the staff saw over time. And, of course, Ed always hoped for the best, which may have clouded his ability to identify when his mother needed more care. I remember pointing out that she seemed increasingly weak after her last battle with a urinary tract infection (UTI). "No, she'll bounce back," Ed nodded. "She always bounces back." With some gentle coaxing, I was able to get Ed to consider what it may be like if she didn't bounce back. "Let's talk to a hospice organization—just in case," I had suggested.

As Dr. Anne Kenny says in her informative book *Making Tough Decisions about End-of-Life Care in Dementia*, "The final stages are known for the loss of ability to fully engage with the environment. This stage may be confusing for family members, as 'good' days with glimmers of independence and function are interspersed with 'bad' days that require assistance for safety or to avoid frustration" (p. 18).

As we discussed in chapter 4, the later stages of the disease are often accompanied by a loss of basic functions of daily life. These losses often go hand in hand with repeated infections or other illnesses, as was the case with Ed's mother's recurring UTIs.

Although I have always made it a point to discuss end-of-life care planning with care partners, not all health care professionals do—and I find this to be unfortunate. End-of-life care is an important continuation of care during life. It may fall to you, the care partner, or the family as a whole to decide when to call a hospice organization. Don't wait for a health care professional at your loved one's senior living community to broach the topic. Instead, ask them about it when you begin to notice that your family member or friend's dementia is progressing. There is no harm in asking about hospice. The only thing that may happen is that it's too early and your friend doesn't qualify for hospice care. You are always free to bring it up at a later date.

How Does End-of-Life Planning Work?

End-of-life planning starts with a conversation, albeit a difficult one. It is best to start having conversations about what you or your loved ones would want at the end of life long before you or they can no longer communicate those wants and needs. This is called advance care planning. I recommend putting these needs in writing, so that when the time comes, there is no confusion or disagreement over what you or someone else wanted. Find out who the person wants to choose as a health care proxy—that is, the person that will be making health care decisions on their behalf. It is always a good idea to have a durable power of attorney signed and ready as someone's dementia progresses. One of the most challenging and upsetting moments in anyone's care journey is when they begin to refuse care, and the family is unable to do anything about it.

The Fives Wishes form, which is easy to use and can take the place of an individual's living will, is available and legally accepted in most states in the United States. The user writes down their preferences regarding life-saving measures, funeral arrangements, organ donation, and more. A form like this saves a person's family from having to make hard choices amongst themselves. Many hospice organizations offer free copies of the Five Wishes form, or you can purchase an inexpensive (usually around $5) copy online.

A POLST is another useful form available and accepted in most states, although some states use a different name for the form. The POLST, short for Physician Orders for Life-Sustaining Treatment, is an advance directive that is completed through a conversation between a person's physician and their family. It identifies a surrogate decision maker and provides information about what a person wants during a medical emergency. A POLST is usually appropriate for a person who expects to die within one year. Care partners for those living with dementia may find it useful to keep their loved one's POLST some-where handy, such as posted on the fridge.

What if a person living with dementia has never discussed their wants and needs regarding spirituality and care for the end of their life? How do you know what they want? Hospice organizations provide plenty of choices and ideas. For example, many hospices offer spiritual counselors of different faiths. If the person you are caring for is religious, it makes sense that they would appreciate a spiritual leader like a pastor or rabbi at their bedside. Many hospices also offer volunteer services, such as musicians who will come play music in a person's room. Hospice can help walk you through the available options and choose a plan that works for you and the person living with dementia.

Putting It into Practice

Writing about the many emotions related to hospice in a journal can be immensely helpful. There is a lot of evidence to support that journaling helps us to process and organize them. Hospice and end-of-life care are stressful topics that many families would prefer to avoid. I encourage you, however, to take a few minutes and write down your thoughts related to the following questions, even if you don't believe it's time to consider hospice for a loved one.

1. What is my biggest fear regarding hospice?

_____

2. What is stopping me from talking to loved ones about hospice?

_____

3. When I hear the word *hospice*, I think of:

_____

4. I know that my loved one would want _____ at the end of their life.

5. At the end of my life, I would want to make sure everyone knows that I _____.

RESOURCES

Five Wishes. 2021. The Five Wishes Advance Directive. https://fivewishes.org/shop/order/product/five-wishes.

Kenny, A. 2018. *Making Tough Decisions about End-of-Life Care in Dementia.* Baltimore: Johns Hopkins University Press.

National Hospice and Palliative Care Organization. 2021. https://www.nhpco.org.

POLST. 2021. National POLST. https://polst.org. POLST forms are portable medical orders or medical orders that travel with the patient. Your state may call it something other than POLST; see the list of variations:

- AzPOLST: Arizona Provider Orders for Life-Sustaining Treatment
- COLST: Clinician Order for Life Sustaining Treatment
- DMOST: Delaware Medical Orders for Scope of Treatment
- IPOST: Iowa Physician Orders for Scope of Treatment
- LaPOST: Louisiana Physician Orders for Scope of Treatment
- MOLST: Medical Orders for Life-Sustaining Treatment
- MOST: Medical Orders for Scope of Treatment
- OkPOLST: Oklahoma Physician Orders for Life-Sustaining Treatment
- PA POLST: Pennsylvania Orders for Life-Sustaining Treatment
- POLST: Physician Orders for Life-Sustaining Treatment
- POST: Physician Orders for Scope of Treatment
- SAPO: State Authorized Portable Orders
- SMOST: Summary of Physician Orders for Scope of Treatment
- TOPP: Transportable Orders for Patient Preferences
- TPOPP: Transportable Physician Orders for Patient Preference
- WyoPOLST: Wyoming Providers Orders for Life-Sustaining Treatment

CHAPTER 34

When There's a Hospital Trip

How to make a hospital trip less stressful

A trip to the hospital always seems to sneak up on families of those living with dementia. It's unexpected and sudden, and usually starts with what is called a *precipitating event*. A precipitating event is an event that leads to a sudden decline in a person's functioning. Examples include falls, strokes, urinary tract infections, dangerous medication interactions, and choking.

Hospital trips are always disorienting for adults living with dementia and their families. Often, people living with dementia return from the hospital more agitated and confused than before they went in. In this chapter, we will discuss how to how to cope with hospital trips and the chaos they can bring.

Precipitating Events

As I said, precipitating events are accidents or sudden illnesses that cause someone to decline. Often, these events send someone to the hospital. According to the National Council on Aging, falls are the leading cause of death in older adults. Every eleven seconds, an older adult is treated in the emergency department for trauma caused by a fall (National Council on Aging).

Ralph had been a resident at our dementia care community for some time. He had been doing well and was considered to be high functioning for an older adult living in a moderate stage of Alzheimer disease. He was very social and friendly, and his family visited him frequently. One day, he tripped on his way to lunch, catching the side of his shoe on the leg of a chair. He crashed to the floor, unable to break his fall.

Because Ralph hit his head and seemed more confused than normal, we didn't hesitate to call 911, requesting that Ralph be evaluated by the paramedics and taken to the hospital. Staff members always evaluate the seriousness of the fall before sending someone to the emergency department, since ER trips can be traumatic for everyone involved. If Ralph had seemed fine and had not hit his head—almost always a reason to send someone to the hospital—we probably would not have sent him out.

It is common in dementia care communities to host a quick morning meeting between staff members of third and first shift, and to include management in that meeting. The team dis-cusses changes in the condition of their residents, including who went out recently. "Going out" is shorthand for going to the hospital or to an emergency department. If the resident who falls is on hospice services, hospice will help determine if the resident should transfer to the hospital. Sending someone to the hospital is usually considered to be a life-saving measure. Individuals who have been admitted to hospice services have decided they no longer want life-saving measures. (For more on hospice, see chapter 33.)

Delirium

Delirium is a sudden onset of confusion brought on by a precipitating event. Delirium should be taken seriously. If a person living with dementia is significantly worse than they were the day before, it can be an indication of delirium. Dementia does not get worse overnight, so any precipitating event needs to be identified and treated.

When someone living with dementia has an accident, they can decline suddenly. This dramatic change is always jarring for the staff and family. In some instances, an individual will have a precipitating event, show significant decline, and then get a little bit better. This "better," though, is not necessarily where their old baseline was, and so their overall decline is evident.

Hospital-induced delirium is also common among people with dementia. Someone will come back from the hospital more confused than when they went in. The causes of hospital-induced delirium differ from person to person, but they are commonly changes in medication, exhaustion, and a sense of being overwhelmed by the sights and sounds of the hospital.

Can someone recover from hospital-induced delirium? The simple answer is yes, but more often than not, it depends. I have watched residents go to the hospital, come back delirious, and then improve back to their baseline. I have also seen residents come back from the hospital delirious, and while the delirium fades, their overall decline remains and then worsens.

The Hospital Trip

Many trips to the hospital trip are preceded by an accident. Once the paramedics have been called, the family or care partner is notified by telephone that their spouse, friend, or family member has had an accident and will be going to the hospital. The family or care partner can meet the person living with dementia at the hospital. At the end of the chapter, I give some tips for making hospital trips less stressful, both for you and for the person living with dementia.

In all cases, remain calm. If you show up at the hospital agitated and stressed, you are going to make it more stressful for the individual you're caring for. In Ralph's case, he was calm and pleasant on his way to the hospital. I don't know what happened when he arrived there, but I do know that his daughter was typically a highly stressed individual. She may have showed up at the hospital tearful and stressed, which in turn made her father feel upset.

I also recommend packing a bag that contains your loved one's personal belongings and their important medical information. While the senior living community may send them to the hospital with some information, it's always good for you to bring that information to the hospital, too. So, be sure you know what medications they are currently taking, the dosages, and how often. Typically, hospitals discharge (written as D/C) some medications and then prescribe or increase the dosages of others. I have found that families are often unaware or surprised by the changes in medications that a hospital physician made. "Wait, I had no idea that dad was prescribed an anti-psychotic!" I have heard families exclaim. "When did that happen?"

> Bailey had declined significantly since her hospital stay. She wasn't her perky, upbeat self. She'd had a hip fracture, a common accident for an older adult. To repair the fracture, Bailey had to undergo an operation. In this operation, as with many intensive operations, the doctors put her under general anesthesia. Now, a week after surgery, she was lethargic, confused, and irritable.

Anesthesia negatively affects older adults more than it does younger people, and it is particularly hard on adults living with dementia. Postoperative cognitive decline/dysfunction (POCD) is more common in people living with dementia. Unlike delirium, which should subside within a week or so of surgery, POCD can affect people for many weeks or months after surgery. Does this mean that people living with dementia should not have general anesthesia? Not necessarily, but before performing a surgery, physicians must take into account a patient's level of cognitive function and current medications when deciding which anesthesia to use (Dementia Australia).

Changes in medication, long stretches spent lying in bed, noises, lights, and constant shuffling of people through hospital rooms do not help the cognition of someone who is already confused. For example, shiny hospital floors can appear to be wet to someone who is cognitively impaired. To ease this confusion, some hospitals offer acute care for the elderly units, known as ACE units. These units designed for older adults who are admitted to the hospital. ACE unit staff are trained to work with the elderly and the cognitively impaired. ACE units tend to look less "hospital-like" than the rest of the hospital, which helps calm agitated patients. Some have activity spaces or offer activity carts to patients living with dementia. Princeton Medical Center in New Jersey places a purple seahorse symbol on the door of patients who are living with dementia. The seahorse designates a person's cognitive impairment without making it obvious to the patient. It's a great idea; staff know which of their patients may need a little extra assistance.

After the Hospital Stay Is Over

I cannot stress this enough: before you and your loved one leave the hospital, know where they are going next. Having worked in many care community settings, I can tell you that it is overwhelming and stressful for the community when we get a brand-new resident without any warning. "Hey, we have so-and-so coming from the hospital today," I would sometimes hear from a nursing supervisor. "Just so you know!" This was never enough information for me, so I cannot imagine how troubling it must be for a person living with dementia and their care partners to navigate leaving the hospital and going to a new, sometimes unfamiliar, place.

Information and honesty are key to having a smooth transition. Care partners must be honest with themselves when moving a person with dementia from a hospital to another location. What does this individual need now? Have their needs changed? Do the hospital physicians expect much improvement? Care partners must also be honest with the community their person is transitioning to. Telling staff at an assisted living community that "Mom will be back to normal in no time," is unfair to everyone, including Mom. Perhaps your mother now requires additional dementia-specific care because her condition has worsened. Shifting a cognitively impaired individual around too much is confusing, unkind, and unhealthy.

Recognize that their condition may have worsened since the hospital stay. As we've discussed, this could be due to a change in medications, hospital-induced delirium, effects of anesthesia, or it could be overall decline stemming from the precipitating event and the trip to the hospital. There is a chance that this new baseline is permanent. There is a chance that they won't "bounce back" to where they were prior to going to the hospital. This is frequently what happens in dementia caregiving. I realize it can be scary, but a precipitating event and a hospital stay can result in a significant decline in your loved one's cognitive function.

Putting It into Practice

Here are some tips for making a hospital trip less stressful.

1. Have your loved one's important medical information readily available, preferably printed out and posted or kept in a location where you can find it. This information may include a do not resuscitate (DNR) order, important contacts and where to reach them, information about their medications and medical history, and anything else you deem important.
2. Have a "go-bag" packed for both you and the person who needs to visit the hospital. This go-bag should include some snacks, a change of clothes, a sweater, and a book or game.
3. Do your best to remain calm. If your loved one is being sent out from their senior living community to the hospital, you can meet them at the hospital when you are able. Take a deep breath and prepare for what will probably be a long wait by their side or in the waiting room.
4. Bring something for your loved one to do in the hospital. If they are staying for

a few days or overnight, there is a good chance they will be both bored and overstimulated. Music and headphones, if they will tolerate headphones, can be a calming option.
5. Communicate to other visitors that your loved one may be disoriented or "the worse for wear" at the hospital, and to not be concerned, or at least not to show concern in front of the person living with dementia.
6. Let the hospital staff know that your loved one is cognitively impaired. This may mean you put a note outside their door. In some places, such as some ACE units, these notifications are readily available.
7. Prepare for what will happen after they leave the hospital. Do they need to go to a skilled nursing facility for rehabilitation? Will they be discharged back your house? To their dementia care community? Have a plan for how and when they will get to that location and who will assist them when they arrive.

RESOURCES

Dementia Australia. 2020. Anesthesia for Older People and People with Dementia. https://www.dementia.org.au/files/helpsheets/Helpsheet-DementiaQandA20-Anaethesia_english.pdf.

Gillick, M. R. 2020. *The Caregiver's Encyclopedia: A Compassionate Guide to Caring for Older Adults.* Baltimore: Johns Hopkins University Press.

National Council on Aging. 2021. Falls Prevention for Older Adults. https://www.ncoa.org/older-adults/health/prevention/falls-prevention.

CHAPTER 35

Final Thoughts and Notes

When I first started working in dementia care, I had only my scholastic experience behind me: the books I'd read, the articles I'd reviewed, experts I'd talked to, workshops I'd attended, and a few internships and volunteer experiences. I was fortunate that I was able to gain that knowledge, but even so, none of it truly prepared me for working in the industry. I learned so much, so quickly, working hands-on with adults living with dementia. I started my blog as I started my first job out of graduate school because there were so many amazing stories and experiences I just had to share with others. I also found myself fielding a lot of big questions on a regular basis—questions that I wasn't 100% sure I had the answers to. It would've been amazing to read a book like this one at that time.

Above all else, I want you to come away from this book with better knowledge about dementia care communication. As you well know, communicating with people living with dementia can be challenging. But by Embracing Their Reality effectively, communication—and all other aspects of caregiving—becomes a bit easier. Let's review my ten best strategies for positive communication, empathy, and understanding.

Ten Strategies for Communication

1. Understand that their world may be different from our world, and that's okay. We want to embrace their reality rather than trying to convince them of things that are true in our reality. Just because their reality is a different shape, it doesn't make it wrong.
2. Don't get hung up on the word "lying." Realize that if you are telling them the facts of their reality, you are doing the best thing for both of you.

3. Use certain wording when asking questions of people living with dementia:

   - "Where do you think they are?" when someone asks you about loved one
   - "Can you help me?" when getting them to do something with you
   - "What do you think about this?" when introducing a baby doll or stuffed animal

4. Knowing the individual on a personal level will always help you live in their reality. Use your listening skills to learn more about where they came from and what their emotional needs are.

5. Offer two or three choices instead of asking open-ended questions like "What do you want to eat for breakfast?" or "What did you do today?"

6. Timeline Confusion is the concept that time isn't linear for people living with dementia. If the individual cannot identify their loved ones, it isn't because they don't know them or love them, it's because these people don't fit on their timeline.

7. Never try to convince someone living with dementia of something. Don't use logic to try to help them understand.

8. No weddings, no funerals, no cemeteries. In other words, don't bring a loved one living with dementia to an event that could be overwhelming. Weddings and funerals can be incredibly stressful, albeit for different reasons. I always say, "no cemeteries" because I don't want a family taking Mom to a cemetery to prove to her that Dad has passed away. If Mom wants to go visit Dad, that's fine, but we never want to use logic to force someone to understand a loved one has died.

9. Avoid reorientation. Remember that there are degrees of reorientation. Just because you aren't taking them to the cemetery doesn't mean it is okay to remind them who died— that's still reorientation.

10. Recognize that their timeline and reality may change, and we must learn to be flexible and change with it. Dementia caregiving is an art form that takes practice and patience to do well.

Bringing It All Together

My hope is that this book provides family members and loved ones of those living with dementia with answers, tips, strategies, and encouragement. The staff and management at care communities should find helpful information in here, too. I wrote this book to provide insight into dementia care communities: the differences among them, the services they provide, who lives there, who works there, and, most of all, how you can make the most of such a community for your friend or family member, residents, and clients.

You now have an idea of what to expect when moving someone into a dementia care community, and I hope this book has eased your mind about that decision. The choice to move someone into a dementia care community is challenging. You will have your doubts, your concerns, and even arguments with yourself and others. Still, you have good reason to hope for the best. You are making a decision that affects both you and your family member, and it can be a beautiful choice.

Dementia care communities exist to provide caregivers with another option. They represent an opportunity to give your family member or friend a better life than they could receive at home. Most families intend to provide the best care possible. But care communities are equipped with all the tools to provide twenty-four-hour physical and emotional care to adults living with dementia. Dementia care communities draw out and preserve from your family member or friend living with dementia the essential qualities that make them human: the ability to love, the desire to learn, and the eagerness to live a meaningful life. Many families are concerned that they are "caging" a loved one when they join a care community. Instead, think of a care community as a place where people living with dementia can be safe and secure from the outside world, while thriving as best they are able to. This is not a terrible thing. They have joined a community with adults their own age and cognitive level, where they have the opportunity to make true friendships.

Perhaps you felt uncomfortable learning that some people living with dementia will kindle new romantic relationships at the community. Although that can be unsettling to think about, try to accept that those living with dementia deserve the opportunity to meet and engage with new people. They deserve the chance to make friends, create relationships, and even have a romantic partner if they so choose. A dementia care community allows for this in a way that home care does not.

Perhaps you worry that your parent, partner, child, or friend will just fade away in a community. Consider that the people who work in dementia care communities are prepared to engage with and entertain the residents. In good communities, there are activities and entertainers designed specifically for people living with dementia. Your dad living with dementia, for example, will not just sit there, bored, on a couch all day.

Remember that your dad living with dementia does not live in the same world that you do. He exists in another reality, a reality where time is confusing and his relationship with it is mixed up. Those living with dementia may live in the world they lived in years ago: where they are working for a living, are still married, and their children are young. At a dementia care community, a person living with dementia has the opportunity to live in that world. All good care communities have a reason for offering baby dolls, realistic-looking stuffed animals, and life-skills stations that resemble things we would see out in the real world.

Consider that you, as a caregiver, can have a better life when your family member or friend lives in dementia care community. Perhaps this feels like a selfish reason to choose a community for someone, but it's a decision that will ensure the best care for yourself and your family member. When I've spoken to caregivers who made the transition, they've often told me that despite the difficulty of the choice, they feel closer with their loved one after the move. Suddenly, they're more than just the caregiver: they're the friend, loved one, partner, or child again. It is difficult to provide the best possible care when you as a caregiver are stressed and unhappy.

Dementia Does Not Have to Be Terrible

Although dementia is distressing, a person who is living with dementia does not have to lead a terrible existence. People living with dementia can live out happy, healthy, and fulfilling lives in care communities. People living with dementia live in a different world than we do—a world with the possibility of being in a much happier place than the real world. Instead of being 90 years old and riddled with physical ailments, a woman living with dementia may believe that she is 30 and still in the prime of her life.

I closed my first book with this story, and I thought about changing it in this book—but I really do love it. I hope you do, as well.

"We had a great time today," Alexis told me as we walked down the hallway.

"Oh, yeah?" I asked. "What were you all doing?"

"My group of gals and I went dancing at this senior community," Alexis said, smiling. "The old folks really seemed to enjoy it, too. They were clapping and laughing and dancing. It was really a beautiful moment, wish you could've been there."

Alexis was living with dementia and lived in our care community. She had been, at one point in her life, a dancer. From what I gathered, she was really quite the star. Alexis had danced all over New York City and on Broadway.

On this particular day, Alexis's mind had convinced her that she had been dancing at a senior living community. This story was funny because she *had* been dancing at a senior community— her own community, where she lived. Alexis had seen the older faces in the crowd as she cruised across the floor, dancing in time to the beat of the accordion player. She had seen the older adults—her friends, her companions—get up and dance with her. Alexis believed that she and her dancing group had volunteered at a senior living community, but in reality she had been dancing on her own dementia care floor.

She regularly regaled us with stories of her younger days, even though they were always told in the present tense. Alexis believed, without a doubt, that she currently lived that life she had loved so very much. She was still a dancer. She was still a young woman—meeting men, laughing, going out, eating fabulous dinners, and engaging in interesting conversation.

She was not an 85-year-old woman who sometimes fell asleep on our activity room couch with no shoes on. Alexis was not a confused woman who needed help showering and organizing her closet. She was not a woman who needed to be escorted to the dining room so she would not forget where it was. Alexis was, in her world, an adventurer living her life to the fullest. And we believed that, too.

———————

Thank You

Thank you for reading my book. I hope that you've empathized as I've retold stories about my residents, and I hope, most of all, that you laughed more than you cried. I hope that you can push away the guilt and anxiety you feel over caregiving, whatever your situation. Know that I think you're doing a great job, just because you finished this book. The fact that you picked up a book about dementia caregiving—when really it's all you think about every day, anyway—means that you are hungry for knowledge and assistance. Your loved one living with dementia will benefit from the lessons you've learned, and you will feel better as you navigate your role as care partner. Congratulations on doing what's best for you both, and thank you for being here.

Best wishes for your health and the health of those you care for,
Rachael

Appendix
Clinical Dementia Rating Scale

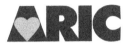 **CLINICAL DEMENTIA RATING SUMMARY**

ID NUMBER:		FORM CODE:	C	D	S	DATE: 06/01/2011
						Version 1.0

ADMINISTRATIVE INFORMATION

0a. Completion Date: ☐☐ / ☐☐ / ☐☐☐☐   0b. Staff ID: ☐☐☐

Month   Day   Year

> **Instructions**: *This form is to be completed by the clinician or other trained health professional based on informant report and neurological exam of the subject. In the extremely rare instances when no informant is available the clinician or other trained health professional must complete this form utilizing all other available information and his/her best clinical judgment. Score only as decline from previous level due to cognitive loss not impairment due to other factors.*

SECTION 1: STANDARD CDR

Please enter scores below.	None 0	Questionable 0.5	IMPAIRMENT Mild 1	Moderate 2	Severe 3
1. MEMORY ___.___	No memory loss, or slight inconsistent forgetfulness.	Consistent slight forgetfulness; partial recollection of events; "benign" forgetfulness.	Moderate memory loss, more marked for recent events; defect interferes with everyday activities.	Severe memory loss; only highly learned material retained; new material rapidly lost.	Severe memory loss; only fragments remain.
2. ORIENTATION ___.___	Fully oriented.	Fully oriented except for slight difficulty with time relationships.	Moderate difficulty with time relationships; oriented for place at examination; may have geographic disorientation elsewhere.	Severe difficulty with time relationships; usually disoriented to time, often to place.	Oriented to person only.

	IMPAIRMENT				
Please enter scores below.	None 0	Questionable 0.5	Mild 1	Moderate 2	Severe 3
3. JUDGMENT & PROBLEM SOLVING ___.___	Solves everyday problems, handles business and financial affairs well; judgment good in relation to past performance.	Slight impairment in these activities.	Moderate difficulty in handling problems, similarities and differences; social judgment usually maintained.	Severely impaired in handling problems, similarities and differences; social judgment usually impaired.	Unable to make judgments or solve problems.
4. COMMUNITY AFFAIRS ___.___	Independent function at usual level in job, shopping, volunteer and social groups.	Life at home, hobbies and intellectual interests slightly impaired.	Unable to function independently at these activities, although may still be engaged in some; appears normal to casual inspection.	No pretense of independent function outside the home; appears well enough to be taken to functions outside the family home.	No pretense of independent function outside the home; appears too ill to be taken to functions outside the family home.
5. HOME & HOBBIES ___.___	Life at home, hobbies and intellectual interests well maintained.	Life at home, hobbies, and intellectual interests slightly impaired.	Mild but definite impairment of function at home; more difficult chores abandoned; more complicated hobbies and interests abandoned.	Only simple chores preserved; very restricted interests; poorly maintained.	No significant function in the home.
6. PERSONAL CARE ___.___	Fully capable of self-care.		Needs prompting.	Requires assistance in dressing, hygiene, keeping of personal effects.	Requires much help with personal care; frequent incontinence.
7. ___.___ STANDARD CDR SUM OF BOXES					
8. ___.___ STANDARD GLOBAL CDR					

Clinical Dementia Rating Form

SECTION 2: SUPPLEMENTAL CDR

	IMPAIRMENT				
Please enter scores below.	None 0	Questionable 0.5	Mild 1	Moderate 2	Severe 3
9. BEHAVIOR, COMPORTMENT AND PERSONALITY ___.___	Socially appropriate behavior.	Questionable changes in comportment, empathy, appropriateness of actions.	Mild but definite changes in behavior.	Moderate behavioral changes, affecting interpersonal relationships and interactions in a significant manner.	Severe behavioral changes, making interpersonal interactions all unidirectional.
10. LANGUAGE ___.___	No language difficulty or occasional mild tip-of-the-tongue.	Consistent mild word finding difficulties; simplification of word choice; circumlocutions; decreased phrase length; and/or mild comprehension difficulties.	Moderate word finding difficulty in speech; cannot name objects in environment; reduced phrase length and/or agrammatical speech; and/or reduced comprehension in conversation and reading.	Moderate to severe impairment in either speech or comprehension; has difficulty communicating thoughts; writing may be slightly more effective.	Severe comprehension deficit; no intelligible speech.
11. ___.___ SUPPLEMENTAL CDR SUM OF BOXES					
12. ___.___ STANDARD & SUPPLEMENTAL CDR SUM OF BOXES					

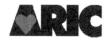

INSTRUCTIONS FOR THE
CLINICAL DEMENTIA RATING (CDR) – SUMMARY;
(CDS) FORM

I. General Instructions

The Clinical Dementia Rating or CDR was developed at the Memory and Aging Project at Washington University School of Medicine in 1979 for the evaluation of staging severity of dementia. The CDR is a five-point scale in which CDR-0 connotes no cognitive impairment, and then the remaining four points are for various stages of dementia:

     0.5 = questionable, or very mild dementia

     1 = mild

     2 = moderate

     3 = severe

The CDR score is derived from information collected from the informant interview as well as the subject interview. The six domains used to construct the overall CDR score are: Memory, Orientation, Judgment and Problem-Solving, Community Affairs, Home and Hobbies, and Personal Care. Each of the domains is rated separately based on the participant's cognitive ability to function in these areas. If the participant is limited in performing activities at home because of physical frailty, this should not affect their scoring on the CDR.

To aid in rating the severity in each of the domains, the CDR table, which shows the six cognitive domains the various severity levels, also provides descriptors for each severity at each box score. These descriptors are meant to be used as guides. The clinician should attempt to distinguish which is the best representation of severity for that particular domain. In situations where the clinician cannot decide between one and two severity levels, the standard rule is to rate a higher severity level. An example would be if memory is between a mild and a moderate severity rating, between a 1 and a 2 box score, and the clinician cannot determine where the best representation is, the rule would be that memory is rated as a 2.

To the degree that the informant is observant and their information is thought to be accurate, the CDR information provides essential information in scoring. This is particularly true because three of the six domains of the CDR (Community Affairs, Home and Hobbies, and Personal Care) are almost entirely dependent upon the informant interview.

The Informant Interview (CDI) and the Subject Interview (CDP) should be completed within 90 days of each other. If more than 90 days has passed between these interviews, it should be noted in notelogs on both forms. Scoring on the CDS should be based primarily on the later form.

II. Detailed Instructions for Each Item

0a.   Enter the date on which the participant was seen in the clinic.

0b.   Enter the staff ID for the person who completed this form.

1.   Memory: It may be difficult to make a distinction between CDR memory score of 2 or 3. CDR-2 says essentially only highly learned material is recalled and new material is rapidly forgotten, while for CDR-3 only fragments of memory remain. CDR-2 level should be assigned to an individual that appears to have a fairly good recall of essential past personal and historical items and may recall some portions of recent events but not the entire event. Someone with CDR-3 level may recall only a few relatively minor items from the past such as where they were born and whether or not they were married.

Instructions for the Clinical Dementia Rating – Summary QxQ   06/01/2011   Page **1** of **2**

2. Items 2-5 are self-explanatory, in conjunction with the online CDR training that is required of all individuals who administer this scale. In general, the items from the CDI and CDP are labeled by section, to assist the examiner in estimating box scores.

6. Personal Care: Personal Care is unique among the six domains in that it does not have a CDR-0.5 score. At the point where the participant requires some help, if only prompting to change clothes, to shave or to groom their hair, that becomes CDR-1 score. If the participant requires no help, is fully independent, then CDR score should be 0. It is important to emphasize to the participant and the informant that we are asking about <u>change</u> in cognitive ability from prior levels of functioning (sometime over the past year, sometimes compared to 10 years previous).

7-8. Item #7 will be auto-calculated by the DMS, which is simply a sum of the box scores from #1-6. Item # 8 (Standard Global CDR) can be calculated at the following website: http://www.biostat.wustl.edu/adrc/ which will be provided in a link from the DMS, based on the individual box scores from the first 6 items.

11-12. Item #11 is simply a sum of #9 and 10 (auto-calculated by DMS), and #12 is the sum of item 7 and item 11.

Instructions for the Clinical Dementia Rating – Summary QxQ   06/01/2011   Page 2 of 2

Index

accidents, 96, 98, 220–21, 222
ACE (acute care for the elderly) units, 223
activities, 119, 121, 133, 171–78; day trips and
     outings, 166–70; ideas for, 173–78; interactive
     programs, 190–91; during move into dementia
     care communities, 151; online sources, 177;
     during visits, 150, 151, 160, 161, 163
activities of daily living (ADLs), 4, 7, 14, 134–35,
     141, 155; safety precautions for, 112–16
activity boxes, 177–78, 183–84
activity directors, 108, 172
acute care for the elderly (ACE) units, 223
adaptive eating utensils, 195, 197, 198
ADLs. See activities of daily living
administrators, 5, 107, 123, 127, 156–57
adult day care, 3, 4, 49, 88, 129–30, 132, 171
advance care planning, 217
aggression, 71–74, 151, 201–4
aging: as dementia risk factor, 7–8; normal
     cognitive decline during, 8, 9, 13–14
agitation, 9, 19, 43, 67, 71–72, 73, 152, 183;
     hospitalization-related, 220, 222, 223;
     sundowning-related, 72–73, 130, 169, 196;
     urinary tract infection–related, 202
alcohol abuse, 18
Alzheimer disease, 6; aphasia in, 79; concurrent
     with vascular dementia, 17; differentiated
     from dementia, 4, 5, 6–7, 8–9, 14; early-onset,
     8; medications for, 29–30; misdiagnosis, 18;
     risk factors, 8, 14; symptoms, 14–15
Alzheimer's Association, 87, 92, 105
American Bar Association, 133
amyloid hypothesis, 30
amyotrophic lateral sclerosis (ALS), 135, 136
anesthesia, 222, 223
anger, 36, 73, 96, 99, 148, 150, 162, 174, 201, 202,
     209
anti-anxiety medications, 26, 27–28
anxiety, 19, 72, 150, 168, 179, 180, 202, 215;
     anti-anxiety medications, 26, 27–28; in
     caregivers, 89, 103–4, 149, 168, 229

aphasia, 15, 78–83
APOE gene, 8
apps/applications, 187–88, 189–91
aquariums, virtual, 190
arguments, 54, 105, 201–2, 227
Aricept (donepezil), 29–30
art/artwork, 93, 109, 180
art therapy, 49
assisted living facilities (ALFs), 3, 4, 119, 125,
     172, 215; cost, 133, 134; direct care in, 141;
     moving to, 94; respite stays, 127–28; therapy
     teams, 134
attorneys, elder law specialists, 132, 133, 136.
     See also durable power of attorney; medical
     power of attorney

baby dolls, 26, 39, 70, 131, 174–76, 177, 179, 227;
     choosing, 184; sources of, 183–84
balance impairment, 181
balloon-popping apps, 190
bathing and showering, 4, 7, 66, 112, 115, 141,
     142, 155, 215; soap and shampoo (toiletries),
     110, 143, 147, 152
behavioral changes, 69, 202; caregiver's
     understanding of, 70–71; determining the
     causes of, 69–77; in frontotemporal dementia,
     15, 16; urinary tract infection–related, 73, 202
beta-amyloid, 30
bill paying, 94, 95, 98
Birthday Gift (improvisational activity), 50
birthday parties, 62, 88, 193–94
body language, 78, 81, 82
boredom, 72, 171
brain, dementia-related damage, 4, 7, 21, 23, 30,
     55, 80, 175, 206, 207, 211; in frontotemporal
     lobar dementia, 15, 16; in LATE encephalopa-
     thy, 18; in Lewy body dementia, 17, 53; in
     vascular dementia, 16
brain imaging, 10
brain trauma, 18
brain tumors, 8, 18

breathing apps, 190
breathing exercises, for stress relief, 91, 93
BRiTE group, 49–51
Brookdale communities, 190–91
bullying, 109, 119, 199
butter knives, 107–8, 110

calendars, 113; activity, 156, 166, 171
caregivers / care partners: caring for oneself, 87–93; definition, 3, 4; emotional needs, 118, 123; how to approach persons with dementia, 71; in independent living communities, 125; involvement in dementia diagnosis, 10–11; isolation from family, 104–5; long-distance, 103–4; paid, 118; positive attitude, 71, 148–50, 149, 179; questions for, 5; shared caregiving duties, 89; stress in, 85, 87–93, 117, 118, 222, 228; unpaid, 132
CDR (Clinical Dementia Rating) scale, 21, 231–32
cemeteries, visits to, 104, 226
cerebrovascular damage, 16
certified nursing assistants (CNAs), 127
cheating, accusations of, 43, 73
children, interactions with, 66, 166, 167, 175
choking, 7, 23, 140, 192, 193, 194, 220
circadian rhythm, 181
Clinical Dementia Rating (CDR) scale, 21, 231–32
clutter, 112, 114, 115, 153
cognitive decline: beta-amyloid in, 30; definition, 7; improvisational techniques for, 49–51; medications for, 9, 29–31; normal aging–related, 8, 9, 13–14; reversible, 8; symptoms, 4
colors, of rooms, 181
communication, 33; during aggressive behavior, 35–83; aphasia, 78–83; during delusions or hallucinations, 52–57; Embracing Their Reality concept, 35–45; between families and dementia care community management, 157; improvisation techniques, 47–51; negative, 104; nonverbal, 78, 80, 82; of personal preferences, 63–68; quizzing in, 43–45; ten best strategies, 225–26; timeline confusion and, 37, 58–62; use of personal names, 45; during visits, 160–64
confabulation, 52, 59, 60
confusion, 52, 55–56, 65–66, 176, 182; delirium-related, 9, 14, 73, 221; differentiated from hallucinations, 55, 56; during hospitalization, 223; urinary tract infection–related, 202
continuing care retirement communities (CCRCs), 3, 128
cooking, 4, 7, 93, 115, 118

costs, of dementia care, 113, 127, 132–37
couples counseling, 105–6
COVID-19 pandemic, 87, 122
cursing, 80

day trips, 166–70
death and dying, with dementia, 22, 23–25, 88, 89–90, 155
decision-making: choices in, 226; for end-of-life care, 24–25, 214–19; frontal lobe function in, 15; impaired, 14, 15, 21, 22
decision-making, by caregivers, 94–100; for moving to a dementia care community, 101–5, 117–23; other family member's involvement, 101, 102, 103; techniques, 95, 98–100
delirium, 9, 14, 73, 221; hospital-induced, 221, 222, 223
delusions, 52, 53, 54, 56, 60
dementia: advanced/late, 21, 22, 217; definition, 6–7, 13; diagnosis / diagnostic tests, 8, 9–12, 17–18, 19; differentiated from Alzheimer disease, 4, 5, 6–7, 8–9, 14; frontotemporal lobar (FTLD), 13, 15–16, 207; information resources about, 91, 92; with Lewy bodies (DLB), 17, 22, 53; media's portrayal, 110; mild/early, 21, 22; moderate/middle, 21–22; most-common causes, 11, 13–19; myths about, 7–9; Parkinson disease–related, 17, 29; prognosis, 7; symptoms, 4, 6–7, 21–22, 29; as terminal illness, 7, 22, 23–25, 88, 89–90, 155; vascular (VaD), 16–17, 207
dementia care: family members' opposition to, 101–6; as imperfect science, 154–59; multiple levels, 128; positive, 41, 42, 104, 126, 174, 179–80, 186; stereotypes, 124
dementia care communities (DCCs), 4–5, 8, 126; adjustment to, 120–21, 152; benefits of, 119–20, 120–21, 158, 227–29; caregiver's joining of, 89; choice of, 5, 122–23, 126, 130–31, 144; decision to transition loved one to, 117–23; definition, 3; direct care in, 141–47; families' expectations, 154–55, 157, 158; families' relationships with staff members, 155–57; frontotemporal dementia residents, 16; inner workings, 154–59; loved one's readiness for, 119–23; mistakes in, 157; mixed units, 109; moving into, 97; myths about, 107–10; relocation from, 200, 201–2; residents' cognitive levels, 109, 120–21; respite stays, 90; safety precautions in, 107–11, 126, 133, 143; social interactions in, 199–213; staff-to-resident ratio, 143–44, 147; timing of move into, 120–22, 130; types, 124–31
Dementia Detective Worksheet, 74–77

dentures, 145
depression, 18, 27, 72, 200, 210
depth perception impairment, 14, 181
*Diagnostic and Statistical Manual of Mental
Disorders (DSM)*, 6
dietary changes, 192–98
dietary factors, in dementia, 30
dietary supplements, 32
direct care, 141–47
direct-care staff members, 155, 156, 177, 180, 215
disagreements, with other residents, 201–2
dishes, modifications, 195, 197, 198
distraction techniques, 38
dolls. *See* baby dolls
Do Not Resuscitate (DNR) orders, 114, 224
door chimes, 115
doors: at-home, locks for, 115; glass, 115;
key-entry, 109–10; secured, 109–10, 118, 119,
133
dressing, 4, 7; assistance with, 141, 145, 155,
232; cross-dressing, 211
drinking, assistance with, 195–96
driving, 4; giving up, 94, 95–97, 98, 99–100
drug therapy. *See* medications
durable medical equipment, 136
durable power of attorney, 103, 217

eating: assistance with, 141, 146–47, 159, 196;
dietary changes, 146, 192–98; difficulty in,
146, 192, 194, 195, 197; environment for, 146,
181; refusal of, 196–97
eating utensils, 107–8, 146, 194, 195; modifications, 195, 197, 198
educational resources, about dementia: for
caregivers, 91–92; for family members, 105–6
elder law, 132, 133, 136
electronic talking medication aids, 28
Embracing Their Reality, 35–46, 48, 61, 174, 225;
approaches to avoid in, 39, 41–45; during
hallucinations, 54–55; during move into
dementia care, 150–51; for prevention of
driving, 96–97; by spouses, 104
emergency action plans, 114
emergency room (ER) trips, 220–21
emotions, effect on memory, 43, 44. *See also
specific emotions*
end-of-life care and planning, 24–25, 214–19
end-stage renal disease, 135
environment: at-home, 112–16; changes to, 65,
66, 90; confusion about stimuli in, 55–56;
dementia-friendly, 179–84; immersive
design, 180
environmental changes, 27
executive directors, 127, 156–57, 158, 159, 202

Exelon (rivastigmine), 29–30
exercise, 67, 88, 89, 93
eye contact, 48, 71

falls, 7, 9, 18, 119, 145, 188; medication-related,
27; as mortality cause, 220; as precipitating
events, 22, 23, 220, 221; risk factors, 27, 119,
182; as traumatic brain injury cause, 18
family counseling, 105–6
family gatherings, 226
family members: education about dementia,
105–6; failure to recognize dementia, 101;
shared caregiving with, 89
FAST. *See* Functional Assessment Staging Tool
fear/fearfulness, 56, 72, 103; hallucination-
related, 54; medications for, 27–28; of other
dementia care residents, 72, 119, 120–21, 151,
203
Feil, Naomi, 35
financial planning, for elder care, 133–34
finger food diet, 194
Five Wishes form, 217–18
flooring, 181–82; in hospitals, 223
floral arrangements, 107, 108
forgetfulness, 14, 21, 43. *See also* timeline
confusion
friendships, 199–200, 227; of caregivers, 88, 89,
103
frontal lobe, 15, 80
frontotemporal degeneration. *See* dementia:
frontotemporal lobar
Functional Assessment Staging Tool (FAST),
20–21, 23
furniture: patterned, 181–82; rearrangement,
65, 66

gait disturbances, 16
Gateway Care Home, 180
GDS. *See* Global Deterioration Scale
glass objects, 108, 115
Global Deterioration Scale (GDS), 21
GPS devices, 188–89
grab bars, 115
grief, 24–25, 88, 94
guilt, 88, 94–100, 103–4, 141–42, 207

habits, 62–66
hallucinations, 4, 7, 17, 52, 53, 55, 56, 73
*Handbook of Alzheimer's Disease and Other
Dementias, The* (Budson and Kowall), 15
handrailings, 115
health care proxies, 103, 217
health insurance, 127, 133, 134, 215. *See also*
Medicaid; Medicare

hippocampus, 18
hoarding behavior, 69, 112
hobbies, 21, 63–64, 192, 232; of caregivers, 91, 92, 93
Hogeweyk senior living community (Netherlands), 180
holidays, 167–68, 176
home: desire to return to, 148, 161–62, 164–65, 167; emotional attachment to, 119–20; safety issues, 112–16, 118–19
home care agencies, 88, 112, 128–29, 136
Home Instead Senior Care, 129
hospice care, 5, 24, 214–19; graduating from, 214–15; hospital transfers during, 221; mealtime assistance in, 146–47
hospitals/hospitalization, 220–24

improvisation techniques, 47–51
impulse control impairment, 15
incontinence, 12, 21, 117–18, 129, 143, 232
incontinence products, 144, 147, 215
independence, loss of, 94–95
independent living communities, 120, 124–25, 128, 134, 141
information processing impairments, 6, 78; improvisational approach, 48, 49
in-home care, 3. See also home care agencies
instrumental activities of daily living (IADLs), 4, 7
interactive programs, 190–91
irritability, 9, 14; delirium-related, 73; sundowning-related, 72
Is It Alzheimer's? (Rabins), 6, 8
It's Never 2 Late (interactive system), 190–91

journaling, 93, 98–99, 218
Joy for All Pets, 177, 184, 191
judgment impairment, 6, 15, 21, 22

kitchen appliances, safety precautions, 115, 119
knives, 107–8

language deficits, 4, 6, 14, 15–16, 21, 81, 82–83
LATE. See limbic-predominant age-related TDP-43 encephalopathy
laundry, 4, 7, 141, 146, 160, 173, 184
Lewy, Fritz Heinrich, 17
Lewy body diseases, 17, 22, 53
LGBTQIA+ community, 205, 210–11
licensed practical nurses (LPAs), 127
life histories, 66, 184
life-limiting illnesses, 215
life-skills stations, 179, 180, 183–84

lighting, 114, 115, 181
limbic-predominant age-related TDP-43 encephalopathy (LATE), 18
liquid or puree diet, 146, 192, 193–94, 198
liquids, intake of, 195–96
listening skills, 37, 38, 47, 48, 49, 226
living wills, 217
locator watches, 188–89
logic, impaired, 14, 41, 42–43, 202, 226
loneliness, 73, 171
long-term care, 3–4, 127; cost, 133, 134; home care agency–based care with, 129. See also adult day care; assisted living facilities; continuing care retirement communities; dementia care communities; home care agencies; long-term nursing care; personal care; respite care/stays; skilled nursing facilities
long-term care insurance, 133–34
long-term memory, 15; loss, 14, 80
long-term nursing care, 3. See also skilled nursing facilities
loss: behavioral effects, 72–73; of control, 73, 74
lost, getting, 118
loved ones: deceased, 35, 38–39, 41–42, 43, 46, 48, 52; problems in identification of, 44, 58–62, 160, 226; timeline confusion about, 37, 58–62, 168, 226
lying, 35, 36, 38, 225

Making Tough Decisions about End-of-Life Care in Dementia (Kenny), 24–25, 217
meals: environment for, 146, 181; music during, 182–83; as outings, 166, 167, 168–69; during visits, 161–62, 163
mechanical soft ("ground") diet, 192–93
Medicaid, 127, 132, 133–34, 135, 215
medical alert systems, 188, 189
medical care, refusal of, 217
medical evaluations, 9, 18, 53, 56
medical history, 11–12, 224
medical power of attorney, 103
Medicare, 127, 132, 135–36
medications: for behavioral symptoms, 69; contraindications to, 27, 28; for dementia, 9, 29–32; during hospitalization, 222–23, 224; interactions, 14, 17, 28; management, 28–29, 30, 31–32; over-the-counter, 28; side effects, 27, 28–29; use of multiple medications, 28, 35
memory, effect of emotions on, 43, 44
memory care communities, 3, 4, 21, 25, 111. See also dementia care communities
memory care directors, 156, 158

memory care units, 8, 125, 127
memory clocks, 188
memory loss, 4, 15, 16–17. *See also* long-term memory: loss; short-term memory loss
mild cognitive impairment (MCI), 9, 14, 49–51
mirrors, 55, 56, 108
mobility deficits, 112, 141, 168–69
mobility devices, 115
moment, being present in, 48, 49
mood, effect of music on, 182
mood changes, 4, 7, 14–15, 202
motion alarms, 115, 119–20
motor coordination difficulties, 16
movement deficits, 7, 15, 16, 195
moving, into dementia care communities, 148–53; catastrophic reactions to, 148, 149, 150–51, 152; checklist for, 152–53; first arrival, 151; planning for, 149–51; positive attitude about, 148–51, 153; visits after, 151–52
multiple sclerosis, 136
music, 81, 181–82, 190–91, 197, 218; apps, 190

Namenda, 29–30
name recall impairment, 4, 8, 9, 60, 68, 160
name tags, 61
National Council on Aging, 220
neurocognitive disorder (NCD), 6–7
neuroleptics (antipsychotics), 27
N-methyl-D-aspartate (NMDA) receptor antagonists, 29–30
noise, 55, 72, 167, 183
notes, 98, 113, 114, 115, 188–89
nurses, 127, 129, 157, 215
nursing homes, 127. *See also* long-term care; skilled nursing facilities

occupational therapists/therapy, 115, 134, 135, 136
oral care, 141, 144–45, 152
orientation, 21, 41, 231, 234
outings, 166–70

pain, 72, 73, 215, 216
painting, 91, 93, 151, 174
palliative care, 5, 216
paranoia, 17
Parkinson disease (PD), 17, 136, 195
Parkinson disease dementia (PDD), 17, 29
PARO the robotic seal, 187, 191
parties, 68, 88, 162, 167–68
patterns, on floors or furniture, 181–82
Penn Medicine, Penn Memory Center, 28
perseveration, 81

personal care, 3, 21, 121, 128, 129, 155, 234, 235; in dementia care communities, 66, 126, 133, 134–35, 158; in hospice, 215. *See also* direct care
personal care communities or homes, 3, 125, 129, 133, 215
personal history, 142
personality, 171; changes, 4, 7; personal preferences and, 63–64
personal names, 71, 142; superlatives or alliterations of, 50–51, 61; timeline confusion about, 60, 61
personal preferences, 63–68, 171, 172; for activities, 172, 176–77; for end-of-life care, 217–18
person-centered care, 63
pets, 176, 215; virtual, 190. *See also* stuffed animals
pet therapy, 176, 215
phrase repetition, 81, 91
physical attacks, 201
physical needs, 117–18, 121, 134; direct care for, 141–47
physical spaces. *See* environment
physical therapists/therapy, 115, 127, 134, 135, 136
plateaus, in dementia, 22
plate guards, 195, 198
pneumonia, 23
POLST (Physician Orders for Life-Sustaining Treatment), 218
positive attitude, 71, 148–50, 179
postoperative cognitive decline/dysfunction (POCD), 222
power of attorney, 94; medical, 103
precipitating events, 23, 220–21, 224
Princeton Medical Center, 223
psychiatric evaluations, 10–11
Psychiatry Online, 6
psychomotor skills, loss of, 21
puree or liquid diet, 146, 192, 193–94, 198
puzzles, 174

questions: in improvisational techniques, 47–48, 49; for new dementia care community residents, 63–64, 66; about personal preferences, 65; for reality orientation, 38–40; wording of, 226
quizzing, 39, 41, 43–45, 61–62

Rabins, Peter (*Is It Alzheimer's?*), 6, 8
Razadyne (galantamine), 29–30
reality, perception of, 55, 61. *See also* Embracing Their Reality

reality orientation. *See* reorientation
reasoning, impaired, 4
redirection techniques, 38
reflex speed impairment, 16
regional team oversight, 156–57
registered nurses (RNs), 127
Reisberg, Barry, 20, 21
relocation, of dementia care community
   residents: for disruptive behavior, 201–2;
   after hospitalization, 223–24
Remember Me Senior Care, 126
reorientation, 41–42, 46, 97, 113, 226
repetitive phrases, 81, 91
research, in dementia, 30–31
respite care/stays, 3, 90, 127–28
restaurants, 168–69, 207
restraints, 72
rigidity, 21
roommates, relationships between, 199–200,
   202–3
routines, importance, 65–66

safety issues/precautions: at-home, 112–16,
   118–19; in dementia care communities,
   107–11, 126, 133, 143
SAGE Advocacy and Services for LGBT Elders,
   211
scissors, 107, 108
second languages, loss of, 79–80
senility, 7
sexual behavior and relationships, 205–13;
   consensual, 205–6, 208, 212; extramarital,
   208–9; family's attitudes toward, 211–12;
   inappropriate, 80, 207–8, 212–13; new,
   209–10, 227; sexual disinhibition, 15,
   208
sexual orientation, 205, 210–11
shape discrimination impairment, 16
short-term memory loss, 7, 14–15, 80
singing, 81, 174, 179, 182–83
"16 Things I Would Want If I Got Dementia,"
   67–68
skilled nursing facilities (SNFs), 3, 4, 5, 121–22,
   127; Medicare coverage, 135–36; therapy
   teams, 134
sleep/bedtime, routines for, 66, 67
sleep cycle, 181
smartphones, apps, 187–88, 189–91
snacks, 146, 195–96
"snowing someone," with medication, 27
social interactions, 199–213
social isolation, 119
social workers, 10, 130, 156, 215

sorting or matching activities, 160, 173,
   177–78
spatial awareness impairment, 16, 55
speech deficits. *See* language deficits
speech-language therapy, 134, 135, 136
staff, 126, 154–59; "agency staff," 158; aggression management role, 202, 203; assistance
   from during visits, 161–62; direct-care,
   155; families' relationships with, 155–57;
   knowledge of patients' personal preferences,
   64–65; ratio to residents, 143–44; regional
   team oversight, 156–57; round-the-clock
   availability, 142; turnover rates, 158
staging, of dementia, 20–25
stair lifts, 115, 189
Steel City Improv Theater, 48
stress: in caregivers, 85, 87–93, 117, 118, 222,
   228; management methods, 88–93; of moving
   into care community, 148, 149; as sundowning cause, 72
stroke, 9, 12, 14, 16, 27, 136, 215, 220
stuffed animals, 26, 39, 70, 153, 174–76, 184, 226,
   227; robotic, 177, 184, 187, 191
sundowning, 9, 72–73, 130, 169, 190, 196
support groups/systems, 87, 89, 90, 91, 92, 103,
   105
swallowing, difficulty with, 146, 192, 194, 197

tablets, apps for, 187–88, 189–91
tasks, step-by-step approach, 48, 49
technology, 114; benefits, 187, 189–91; problems
   in relying on, 187–89
terminal illness, dementia as, 7, 22, 23–25, 88,
   89–90, 155
theft, 201; accusations of, 43, 46, 71, 73, 201;
   prevention, 110
thinking, impaired, 4, 14
timeline confusion, 37, 58–62, 168, 226,
   228–29
toileting, 70–71, 115, 141, 143–44
toiletries, 110, 143, 145, 147, 152
toothbrushes, 145, 152
toy animals. *See* stuffed animals
traumatic brain injury (TBI), 18
tremors, 16, 195

University of Pennsylvania Health System,
   Penn Memory Center, 10
University of Pittsburgh, Alzheimer Disease
   Research Center, 28
urinary tract infections (UTIs), 20, 23, 52, 73,
   195–96, 202, 216, 220; as cause of delirium or
   hallucinations, 9, 14, 53, 73

validation therapy, 35, 38

vascular cognitive impairment. *See* dementia: vascular

Veterans' Health Administration, 215

violence, threats of, 201, 203

vision, impaired, 55, 181

visits, 151–52, 160–65, 190; exiting from, 148, 160, 161–65

visual perception, impaired, 6, 14, 16, 55, 181, 182

vitamins, 18

walking impairment, 16, 21

wheelchairs, 24, 71, 121, 124, 136, 167

Whose Line Is It Anyway?, 47

Wright, Chris, 48